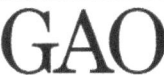

I0426015

April 2012

WORKPLACE SAFETY AND HEALTH

Multiple Challenges Lengthen OSHA's Standard Setting

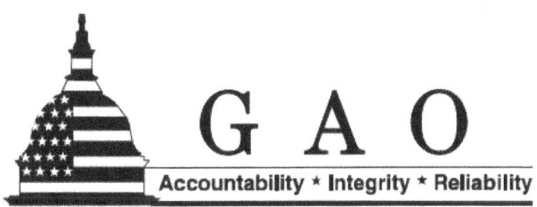

GAO

Accountability ★ Integrity ★ Reliability

GAO
Accountability * Integrity * Reliability
Highlights

Highlights of GAO-12-330, a report to congressional requesters

WORKPLACE SAFETY AND HEALTH

Multiple Challenges Lengthen OSHA's Standard Setting

Why GAO Did This Study

Occupational safety and health standards are designed to help protect about 130 million public and private sector workers from hazards at more than 8 million U.S. worksites. Questions exist concerning how long it takes OSHA to issue its standards. GAO was asked to examine: (1) the time OSHA takes to develop and issue safety and health standards and the key factors that affect these time frames, (2) alternatives to the typical standard-setting process available for OSHA to address urgent hazards (3) whether other regulatory agencies' rulemaking offers insight into OSHA's challenges with setting standards, and (4) ideas from occupational safety and health experts and agency officials for improving OSHA's process. GAO analyzed standards issued by OSHA between 1981 and 2010, interviewed subject matter experts and agency officials at OSHA and two similar federal regulatory agencies and offices, and reviewed the standard-setting process at OSHA and the comparison agencies and offices.

What GAO Recommends

To streamline OSHA standards development, GAO recommends that OSHA and NIOSH more consistently collaborate on researching occupational hazards, so that OSHA can more effectively leverage NIOSH expertise in determining the needs for new standards and developing them. Both agencies agreed with the recommendation.

View GAO-12-330. For more information, contact Revae Moran at (202) 512-7215 or moranr@gao.gov.

What GAO Found

Between 1981 and 2010, the time it took the Department of Labor's Occupational Safety and Health Administration (OSHA) to develop and issue safety and health standards ranged widely, from 15 months to 19 years, and averaged more than 7 years. Experts and agency officials cited increased procedural requirements, shifting priorities, and a rigorous standard of judicial review as contributing to lengthy time frames for developing and issuing standards. For example, they said that a shift in OSHA's priorities toward one standard took attention away from several other standards that previously had been a priority.

In addition to using the typical standard-setting process, OSHA can address urgent hazards by issuing emergency temporary standards, directing additional attention to enforcing relevant existing standards, and educating employers and workers about hazards. However, OSHA has not issued an emergency temporary standard since 1983 because it has found it difficult to compile the evidence necessary to meet the statutory requirements. Instead, OSHA focuses on enforcement and education when workers face urgent hazards. For example, OSHA can enforce the general requirement of the Occupational Safety and Health Act of 1970 (OSH Act) that employers provide a workplace free from recognized hazards, as it did in 2009 when it cited a major retail employer after one of its workers was crushed to death by uncontrolled holiday crowds. To educate employers and workers, OSHA coordinates and funds on-site consultations and publishes information on matters as diverse as safe lifting techniques for nursing home workers and exposure to diacetyl, a flavoring ingredient used in microwave popcorn linked to lung disease among factory workers.

Experiences of other federal agencies that regulate public or worker health hazards offer limited insight into the challenges OSHA faces in setting standards. For example, officials with the Environmental Protection Agency noted that certain Clean Air Act requirements to set and regularly review standards for specified air pollutants have facilitated that agency's standard-setting efforts. In contrast, the OSH Act does not require OSHA to periodically review and update its standards. Officials with the Mine Safety and Health Administration noted that their standard-setting process benefits from both the in-house knowledge of its inspectors, who inspect every mine at least twice yearly, and a dedicated mine safety research group within the National Institute for Occupational Safety and Health (NIOSH), a federal research agency that makes recommendations on occupational safety and health. OSHA must rely on time-consuming site visits for hazards information and has not consistently coordinated with NIOSH to engage that agency's expertise on occupational hazards.

Experts and agency officials identified several ideas that could improve OSHA's standard-setting process. While some of the changes, such as improving coordination with other agencies to leverage expertise, are within OSHA's authority, others call for significant procedural changes that would require amending existing laws. For example, some experts recommended a statutory change that would allow OSHA to revise a group of outdated health standards at the same time, using industry consensus standards as support rather than having to analyze each hazard individually.

_____ United States Government Accountability Office

Contents

Letter		1
	Background	3
	OSHA'S Standard-Setting Time Frames Vary Widely and Are Influenced by the Many Procedural Requirements and Other Factors	7
	OSHA has Authority to Address Urgent Hazards through Emergency Temporary Standards, Enforcement, and Education	20
	Other Regulatory Agencies' Experiences Offer Limited Insight into OSHA's Challenges	26
	Experts Suggested Many Ideas to Improve OSHA's Standard-Setting Process, Including More Interagency Coordination and Statutory Deadlines	30
	Conclusions	37
	Recommendation for Executive Action	38
	Agency Comments	38

Appendix I	Objectives, Scope, and Methodology	41

Appendix II	Selected Procedural Requirements for Federal Rulemaking	44

Appendix III	Comments from the Department of Labor	46

Appendix IV	Comments from the Department of Health and Human Services	48

Appendix V	GAO Contact and Staff Acknowledgments	50

Tables		
	Table 1: Significant OSHA Safety and Health Standards Finalized between 1981 and 2010	8
	Table 2: Selected Procedural Requirements for Federal Rulemaking	44

Figures

Figure 1: Significant OSHA Safety Standards Timeline 10
Figure 2: Significant OSHA Health Standards Timeline 11
Figure 3: Steps in a Typical OSHA Standard-Setting Process 13

Abbreviations

APA	Administrative Procedure Act
EPA	Environmental Protection Agency
MSHA	Mine Safety and Health Administration
NIOSH	National Institute for Occupational Safety and Health
OMB	Office of Management and Budget
OSHA	Occupational Safety and Health Administration
OSH Act	Occupational Safety and Health Act of 1970
PEL	Permissible exposure limit

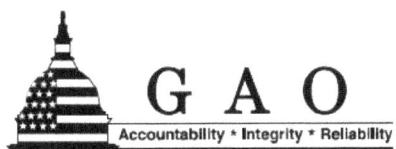

April 2, 2012

Congressional Requesters

Workplace safety and health standards are designed to help protect over 130 million public and private sector workers from hazards at more than 8 million worksites in the United States. Under the Occupational Safety and Health Act of 1970 (OSH Act), as amended,[1] the Department of Labor's (Labor) Occupational Safety and Health Administration (OSHA) issues and enforces occupational safety and health standards, which have been credited with helping prevent thousands of work-related deaths, injuries, and illnesses. For example, OSHA's "lockout/tagout" safety standard requires employers to install devices ensuring that heavy machinery cannot be turned on while being cleaned or repaired. In a 2000 review, OSHA attributed a 55 percent reduction in machinery-related fatalities at 10 steel-producing companies between 1990 and 1997 to the provisions in this standard. However, some occupational safety and health experts have raised questions concerning whether the agency's approach to developing standards is overly cautious, slowing the process and resulting in too few standards being issued. Others counter that the process is intentionally deliberative to balance protections provided for workers with the burden imposed on employers in complying with the standards. Further, over the past 30 years, various presidential executive orders and federal statutes, such as the Regulatory Flexibility Act, have added new procedural requirements for regulatory agencies, resulting in multiple and sometimes lengthy steps OSHA and other agencies must follow. In addition, OSHA's authority covers nearly all U.S. industries, which requires OSHA staff to be familiar with a broad range of processes, equipment, and chemicals used at worksites.

We were asked to review: (1) the time taken by OSHA to develop and issue occupational safety and health standards and the key factors that affect these time frames, (2) alternatives to the typical standard-setting process that are available for OSHA to address urgent hazards, (3) whether rulemaking at other regulatory agencies offers insight into OSHA's challenges with setting standards, and (4) ideas that have been

---

[1]Pub. L. No. 91-596, 84 Stat. 1590, codified as amended at 29 U.S.C. §§ 553, 651-78.

suggested by occupational safety and health experts for improving the process.

To determine how long it takes OSHA to develop and issue occupational safety and health standards, we analyzed new standards and substantive updates to standards finalized between calendar years 1981 and 2010 and identified as significant by the agency. We chose this time frame because it spans multiple executive administrations and changes in congressional leadership. Also, several statutes, executive orders, and key court decisions affecting OSHA's standard-setting process became effective after 1980. To identify the key factors affecting OSHA's time frames for issuing standards and ideas for improving OSHA's standard-setting process, we conducted semistructured interviews with current and former Labor officials and occupational safety and health experts and analyzed their responses. We selected these experts based on our research and the recommendations of other experts. We also reviewed relevant federal laws, regulations, and executive orders, and interviewed officials from the Office of Management and Budget (OMB), to determine the required steps in the standard-setting process and how those requirements affect the time it takes OSHA to develop and issue standards. To identify alternatives to the typical standard-setting process available for OSHA to address urgent hazards, we reviewed relevant federal laws and interviewed current OSHA staff and attorneys from Labor's Office of the Solicitor. We also analyzed relevant agency documentation that Labor officials provided. To determine whether rulemaking at other regulatory agencies offers insight into OSHA's challenges with setting standards, we explored the regulatory process at selected federal regulatory agencies and offices. Through semistructured interviews with policy and program officials at the Environmental Protection Agency (EPA) and at the Mine Safety and Health Administration (MSHA), we learned about challenges each agency faces when developing and issuing similar regulations and factors that affect their time frames. Through our interviews with current and former OSHA officials and experts representing both workers and employers, we identified six ideas for improvement that could expedite or otherwise improve OSHA's standard-setting process. For more information on our objectives, scope, and methodology, see appendix I.

We conducted this performance audit from February 2011 to April 2012 in accordance with generally accepted government auditing standards. Those standards require that we plan and perform the audit to obtain sufficient, appropriate evidence to provide a reasonable basis for our findings and conclusions based on our audit objectives. We believe that the evidence obtained provides a reasonable basis for our findings and conclusion based on our audit objectives.

Background

Basics of the Federal Rulemaking Process

The basic process by which all federal agencies typically develop and issue regulations is set forth in the Administrative Procedure Act (APA)[2] and is generally known as the rulemaking process.[3] Rulemaking at most regulatory agencies follows the APA's informal rulemaking process, also known as "notice and comment" rulemaking, which generally requires agencies to publish a notice of proposed rulemaking in the *Federal Register*, provide interested persons an opportunity to comment on the proposed regulation, and publish the final regulation, among other things.[4] Agencies may also take other actions to gather information during the rulemaking process; for example, agencies may hold a public meeting to allow stakeholders to discuss specific aspects of the proposed regulation. Under the APA, a person adversely affected by an agency's rulemaking is generally entitled to judicial review of that new rule. For regulations developed and issued using the APA's notice and comment rulemaking process, the court may invalidate a regulation if it finds it to be "arbitrary, capricious, an abuse of discretion, or otherwise not in accordance with law," sometimes referred to as the arbitrary and capricious test.[5]

---

[2]Pub. L. No. 79-404, 60 Stat. 237 (1946), codified in 1966 in scattered sections of title 5, United States Code. Agencies may follow additional or alternative procedures if certain exceptions apply, or when required by other statutes. The next section of this report discusses in more detail the process required by the OSH Act for developing and issuing occupational safety and health standards.

[3]The APA defines a rule as "the whole or part of an agency statement of general or particular applicability and future effect designed to implement, interpret, or prescribe law or policy or describing the organization, procedure, or practice requirements of an agency." 5 U.S.C. § 551(4). For this report, we use the terms rule and regulation interchangeably.

[4]5 U.S.C. § 553. The APA also provides for formal rulemaking in certain cases, typically when rules are required by statute to be made on the record after an opportunity for an agency hearing. Formal rulemaking includes a trial-type hearing, and if challenged in court, the resulting rule will be struck down if unsupported by substantial evidence.

[5]5 U.S.C. §§ 702, 706(2)(A).

In addition to the APA requirements, federal agencies typically must comply with requirements imposed by certain other statutes and executive orders. Some of the relevant laws include the Paperwork Reduction Act and the Regulatory Flexibility Act, which were both enacted in 1980;[6] the Congressional Review Act, enacted in 1996;[7] and the Information Quality Act, enacted in 2000.[8] (See app. II for an overview of requirements that commonly apply to OSHA standard setting.) In accordance with various presidential executive orders, agencies work closely with staff from OMB's Office of Information and Regulatory Affairs, who review draft regulations and other significant regulatory actions prior to publication.[9] Most of the additional requirements that affect OSHA standard setting were established in 1980 or later.

Agencies can supplement the notice and comment procedure for developing regulations through a process called "negotiated rulemaking." Through this process, the agency convenes a negotiated rulemaking committee, generally composed of representatives of the agency and the various interest groups to be affected by a potential regulation, before developing and issuing the proposed rule. If the committee comes to an agreement on the content of a potential regulation, the agency may use it as the proposed rule. However, any agreement by the negotiated rulemaking committee is not binding on the agency or interest groups

---

[6]Paperwork Reduction Act of 1980, Pub. L. No. 96-511, 94 Stat. 2812, codified as amended at 44 U.S.C. §§ 3501-20 and Regulatory Flexibility Act, Pub. L. No. 96-354, 94 Stat. 1164 (1980), codified as amended at 5 U.S.C. §§ 601-12.

[7]Subtitle E of the Small Business Regulatory Enforcement Fairness Act of 1996 is known as the Congressional Review Act, Pub. L. No. 104-121, § 251, 110 Stat. 847, 868-74, codified at 5 U.S.C. §§ 801-808.

[8]Section 515 of the Consolidated Appropriations Act, 2001 is known as the Information Quality Act. Pub. L. No. 106-554, § 515, 114 Stat. 2763, 2763A-153 to 2763A-154 (2000) (44 U.S.C. 3516 note). The law is also known as the Data Quality Act.

[9]A regulatory action is "significant" if it will (1) have an annual effect on the economy of $100 million or more or adversely affect in a material way the economy, a sector of the economy, productivity, competition, jobs, the environment, public health or safety, or state, local, or tribal governments or communities; (2) create a serious inconsistency or otherwise interfere with an action taken or planned by another agency; (3) materially alter the budgetary impact of entitlements, grants, user fees, or loan programs or the rights and obligations of the recipients; or (4) raise novel legal or policy issues arising out of legal mandates, the President's priorities, or the principles set forth in Executive Order 12866. Exec. Order No. 12866, 58 Fed. Reg. 51,735 (Sept. 30, 1993). The principles, structures, and definitions established in Executive Order 12866 were reaffirmed by Executive Order 13563, 76 Fed. Reg. 3821 (Jan. 18, 2011).

represented on the committee. Negotiated rulemaking does not replace any procedures required by the APA; rather, it can be used to help reach agreement among the members of the committee on the content of a proposed regulation, and according to proponents, it may help decrease the likelihood of subsequent litigation over the regulation.[10]

Legal Framework and Staffing for OSHA's Standard-Setting Process

OSHA administers the OSH Act, which was enacted to help assure, so far as possible, safe and healthful working conditions for the nation's workers.[11] Section 6(b) of the act authorizes the Secretary of Labor to "promulgate, modify, or revoke any occupational safety or health standard" when he or she determines that doing so would serve the objectives of the OSH Act.[12] Occupational safety and health standards are a type of regulation and are defined as standards that require "conditions, or the adoption or use of one or more practices, means, methods, operations, or processes, reasonably necessary or appropriate to provide safe or healthful employment and places of employment."[13] Section 6(b) of the act also specifies the procedures by which OSHA must promulgate, modify, or revoke its standards. These procedures include publishing the proposed rule in the *Federal Register*, providing interested persons an opportunity to comment, and holding a public hearing upon request.

Section 6(a) of the OSH Act directed the Secretary of Labor (through OSHA) to adopt any national consensus standards or established federal standards as safety and health standards within 2 years of the date the

---

[10]For more details about the federal negotiated rulemaking framework, see 5 U.S.C. §§ 561-570a.

[11]Pub. L. No. 91-596, § 2, 84 Stat. 1590 (1970).

[12]Codified at 29 U.S.C. § 655(b).

[13]29 U.S.C. § 652(8). Throughout this report we will use the term "OSHA standards" to mean "occupational safety and health standards." OSHA standards address both health and safety hazards. Private employers and most federal employers generally must comply with OSHA standards. Although state and local government employers are not subject to OSHA standards, states that operate their own OSHA-approved occupational safety and health programs are required to include state and local government employers, and state standards must be at least as effective as OSHA standards.

OSH Act went into effect.[14] In general, national consensus standards are safety and health standards that a nationally recognized standards-producing organization, such as the National Fire Protection Association, adopts after reaching substantial agreement among those who will be affected, including businesses, industries, and workers.[15] Unlike OSHA's standards, which are mandatory, employers may choose whether to voluntarily follow national consensus standards. The OSH Act specified that OSHA set standards under section 6(a) without following OSHA's typical standard-setting procedures or the APA, including provisions for public comment. Indeed, according to an OSHA publication, hundreds of requirements in current OSHA standards make reference to or are based on about 200 consensus standards, but the OSH Act does not explicitly require OSHA to ensure that these standards are kept up to date.[16] The vast majority of these standards have not changed since originally adopted, despite significant advances in technology, equipment, and machinery over the past several decades. When a federal agency decides to develop a rule, it is generally required by the National Technology Transfer and Advancement Act of 1995 to use technical standards developed or adopted by voluntary consensus standards bodies, where appropriate, except when doing so is inconsistent with

---

[14]Codified at 29 U.S.C. § 655(a). The OSH Act defines an "established Federal standard" as any operative occupational safety and health standard established by any federal agency or contained in any Act of Congress that was in effect on the date of enactment of the OSH Act. 29 U.S.C. § 652(10). Prior to the enactment of the OSH Act, other federal laws included provisions designed to protect workers' safety and health, such as the 1936 Walsh-Healey Act. OSHA included many existing federal standards in the standards it promulgated under section 6(a) of the OSH Act.

[15]For purposes of section 6(a) of the OSH Act, a national consensus standard must have been (1) adopted and promulgated by a nationally recognized standards-producing organization using such procedures that the Secretary of Labor can determine that interested and affected persons reached substantial agreement on its adoption, (2) formulated in a manner which afforded an opportunity for diverse views to be considered, and (3) designated as a national consensus standard by the Secretary of Labor after consultation with other appropriate federal agencies. 29 U.S.C. § 652(9).

[16]However, the Regulatory Flexibility Act requires that agencies develop a plan for periodic review of rules that have or will have a significant economic impact upon a substantial number of small entities to determine whether changes should be made to minimize such impact. 5 U.S.C. § 610. In addition, Executive Order 13563 requires agencies to develop a plan for periodically reviewing existing significant regulations to determine whether they should be modified so as to make the agency's regulatory program more effective or less burdensome. 76 Fed. Reg. 3821 (Jan. 18, 2011).

applicable law or otherwise impractical.[17] Under the OSH Act, if OSHA issues a rule that differs substantially from an existing national consensus standard, the agency must publish in the *Federal Register* an explanation of why its rule will better effectuate the purposes of the OSH Act than the national consensus standard.[18]

OSHA's Directorate of Standards and Guidance, working with staff from other Labor offices, leads the agency's standard-setting process. These staff explore the appropriateness and feasibility of developing standards to address workplace hazards that are not covered by existing standards. Once OSHA initiates such an effort, an interdisciplinary team typically composed of at least five staff focus on that issue.[19]

OSHA'S Standard-Setting Time Frames Vary Widely and Are Influenced by the Many Procedural Requirements and Other Factors

OSHA's Time Frames for Developing and Issuing Standards Vary

We analyzed the 58 significant health and safety standards that OSHA issued between 1981 and 2010 and found that the time frames for developing and issuing them ranged from 15 months to about 19 years (see table 1).[20] At any given point during this period, OSHA staff worked

---

[17]Pub. L. No. 104-113, § 12(d), 110 Stat. 775, 783 (15 U.S.C. § 272 note). If agencies do not use such consensus standards, the law further requires that agency heads provide an explanation to OMB of the agency's reasons.

[18]29 U.S.C. § 655(b)(8).

[19]Teams are usually composed of several staff members from the Directorate of Standards and Guidance, and at least one staff person each from the Office of the Solicitor, the Directorate for Evaluation and Analysis, and the Directorate of Enforcement Programs.

[20]We included in our review standards that OSHA considered to be important or a priority, including but not limited to standards that met the definition of "significant" under Executive Order 12866.

GAO-12-330 Workplace Safety and Health

to develop standards that eventually became final, represented in the table below. On average, OSHA took a total of about 93 months (7 years, 9 months) to develop and issue these standards. After the agency published the proposed standard, it took an average of about 39 months (3 years, 3 months) to finalize the standard. The majority of these standards—47 of the 58—were finalized between 1981 and 1999. In addition to these final standards, OSHA staff have also worked to develop standards that have not yet been finalized. For example, according to agency officials, OSHA staff have been working on developing a silica standard since 1997, a beryllium standard since 2000, and a standard on walking and working surfaces since 2003.[21]

Table 1: Significant OSHA Safety and Health Standards Finalized between 1981 and 2010

Decade/year	Number of standards finalized[a]	Average number of months from initiation to final rule[b]	Average number of months from proposed rule to final rule
1980s	24	70	30
1990s	23	118	50
2000s	10	91	36
2010	1	—[c]	—[c]
Overall	58	93	39

Source: GAO analysis of *Federal Register*.

[a]For the purposes of this analysis, we considered a standard to have been finalized on the date it was published in the *Federal Register* as a final rule.

[b]For the purposes of this analysis, we considered a standard to be initiated on the date OSHA publicly indicated initiating work on the standard in the *Federal Register*, by publishing a Request for Information or Advance Notice of Proposed Rulemaking. In cases where OSHA mentioned neither of these in the final rule, we used the date the standard first appeared on OSHA's semiannual regulatory agenda.

[c]Because only one standard was finalized in 2010, we did not list the average number of months. However, the overall calculations include the 2010 standard.

---

[21]Agency officials told us that OSHA issued a proposed standard on beryllium in 1975, but it was never issued as a final rule. Staff started collecting information on beryllium again in 2000. In addition, they told us that a 2010 proposed rule on walking and working surfaces replaced an outdated proposed rule from 1990 that was never issued as a final rule because of other regulatory priorities.

We found that the time it takes OSHA to develop and issue standards varied over the 30-year period and by the type of standard. First, as shown in table 1, it took OSHA about 70 percent longer, on average, to finalize standards in the 1990s than it took during the 1980s, and about 30 percent longer than during the 2000s. While we were not able to determine the reason for this through our analysis, it demonstrates that there is no clear trend of OSHA developing and issuing standards more or less quickly over time. Second, we found that it took OSHA longer to develop and issue safety standards than health standards—an average of about 8 years, 6 months for safety standards compared with about 6 years, 4 months for health standards—even though several experts to whom we spoke stated that health standards are more difficult for OSHA to issue than safety standards (see figs. 1 and 2 for a depiction of the timelines for safety and health standards issued between 1981 and 2010).[22] Part of this difference may be explained by the fact that a larger portion of the health standards (6 of 23, compared with only 3 of 35 safety standards) were standards for which Congress or the courts articulated time frames for their issuance or development.

---

[22]The number of standards collectively depicted in figures 1 and 2 does not add to 58 because some standards went through substantive revisions and are depicted in the same row.

Figure 1: Significant OSHA Safety Standards Timeline

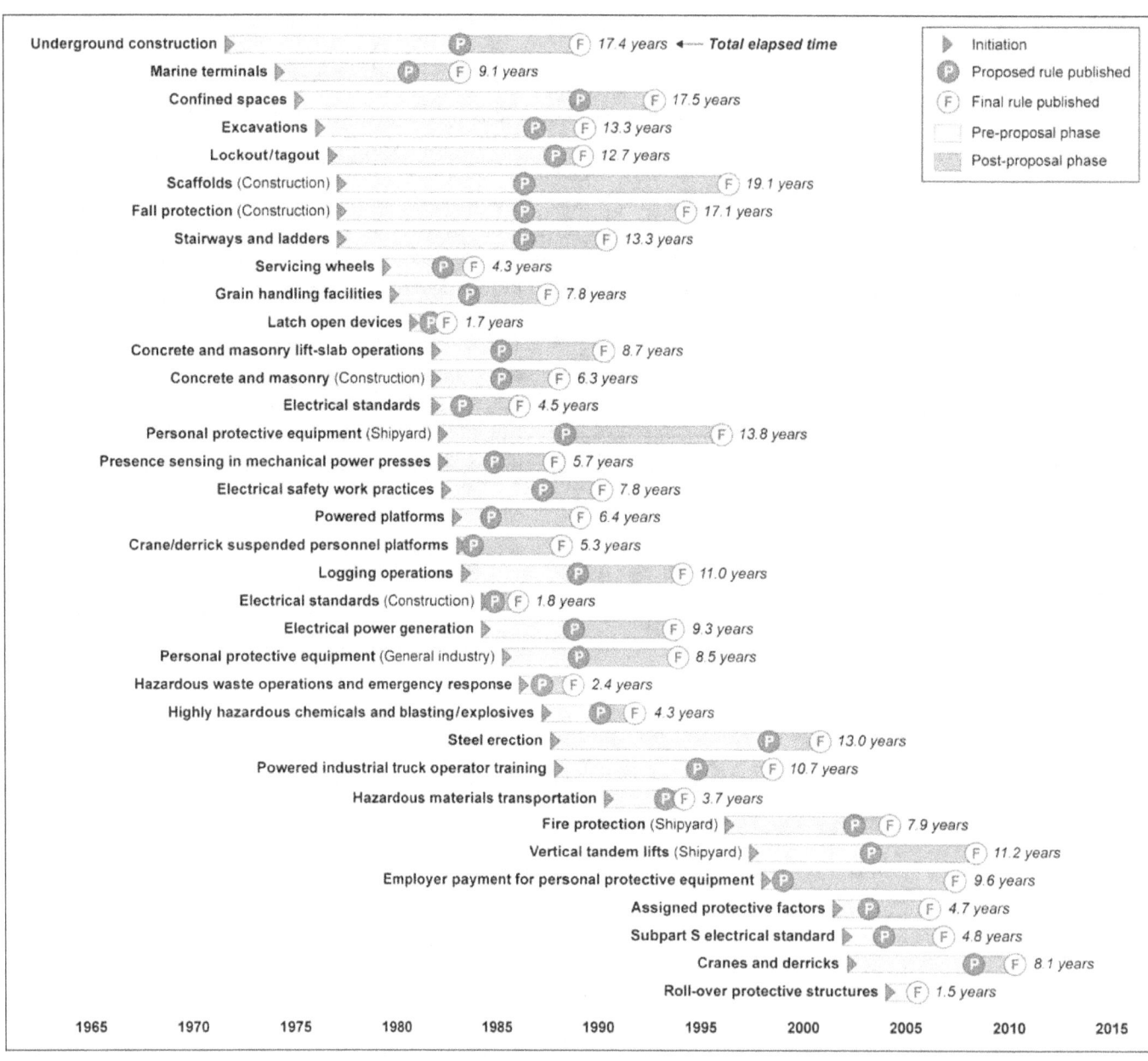

Sources: GAO analysis of interviews with agency officials and *Federal Register* notices.

Note: For the purposes of this analysis, we considered a standard to be initiated on the date OSHA publicly indicated initiating work on the standard in the *Federal Register*, by publishing a Request for Information or Advance Notice of Proposed Rulemaking. In cases where OSHA mentioned neither of these in the final rule, we used the date the standard first appeared on OSHA's semiannual regulatory agenda. We considered a standard to be finalized on the date it was published in the *Federal Register* as a final rule.

Figure 2: Significant OSHA Health Standards Timeline

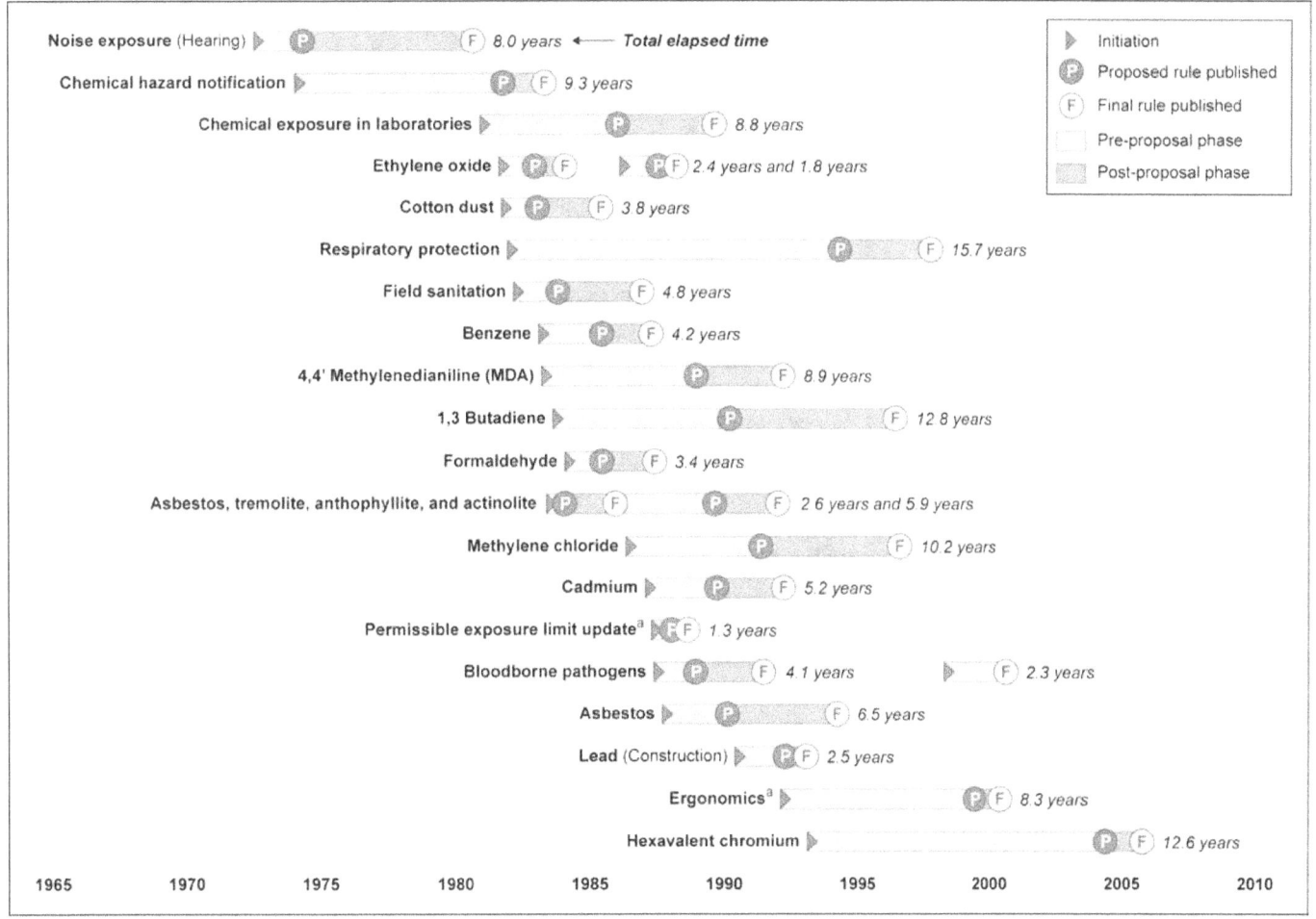

Sources: GAO analysis of interviews with agency officials and *Federal Register* notices

Note: For the purposes of this analysis, we considered a standard to be initiated on the date OSHA publicly indicated initiating work on the standard in the *Federal Register*, by publishing a Request for Information or Advance Notice of Proposed Rulemaking. In cases where OSHA mentioned neither of these in the final rule, we used the date the standard first appeared on OSHA's semiannual regulatory agenda. We considered a standard to be finalized on the date it was published in the *Federal Register* as a final rule.

[a]These two health standards were wholly invalidated either by court decision or congressional action. Parts of other standards may have been invalidated but such analysis is beyond the scope of our review.

GAO-12-330 Workplace Safety and Health

Increased Number of Procedural Requirements, Shifting Priorities, and the High Standard of Judicial Review Cited as Lengthening OSHA's Standard-Setting Process

Experts and agency officials frequently cited the increased number of procedural requirements established since 1980, shifting priorities, and the relatively high standard of judicial review required for OSHA standards as factors that lengthen OSHA's time frames for developing and issuing standards. In addition to these primary factors, several of the experts and agency officials also noted two secondary factors affecting the standard-setting process: significant data challenges and an institutional apprehension about setting standards in the wake of adverse court decisions. We have characterized these as secondary factors because they are both related to the three primary factors.

Increased Number of Procedural Requirements

Experts and agency officials indicated that the increased number of procedural requirements affects standard-setting time frames because of the complex requirements for OSHA to demonstrate the need for standards. Experts and agency officials named a variety of statutes and executive orders that have imposed an increasing number of procedural requirements on OSHA since 1980.

The process for developing and issuing standards is complex and directed by multiple procedural requirements. According to Labor staff, agency consideration of a new standard can be the result of information OSHA receives from stakeholder petitions; occupational safety and health entities, such as the National Institute for Occupational Safety and Health (NIOSH) and the U.S. Chemical Safety and Hazard Investigation Board; OSHA's enforcement efforts; or staff research (see fig. 3).[23] To publicly signal OSHA's intent to pursue development of a new safety or health standard, OSHA typically publishes a Request for Information or an Advance Notice of Proposed Rulemaking on the topic in the Federal Register. In this report, we refer to these events as "initiation." OSHA also signals the beginning of standard-setting efforts by placing the issue on its regulatory agenda.[24] However, OSHA can stop the standard-setting

---

[23]NIOSH is a federal agency located within the U.S. Department of Health and Human Services' Centers for Disease Control. It conducts research and makes recommendations on occupational safety and health. The U.S. Chemical Safety and Hazard Investigation Board is an independent federal agency charged with investigating industrial chemical accidents.

[24]Agencies publish a semiannual regulatory agenda of all regulations under development or review, as required by Executive Order 12866 and OMB guidance. 58 Fed. Reg. 51,735 (Sept. 30, 1993).

process either informally—by ceasing to actively work on the standard—or through a public announcement.

Figure 3: Steps in a Typical OSHA Standard-Setting Process

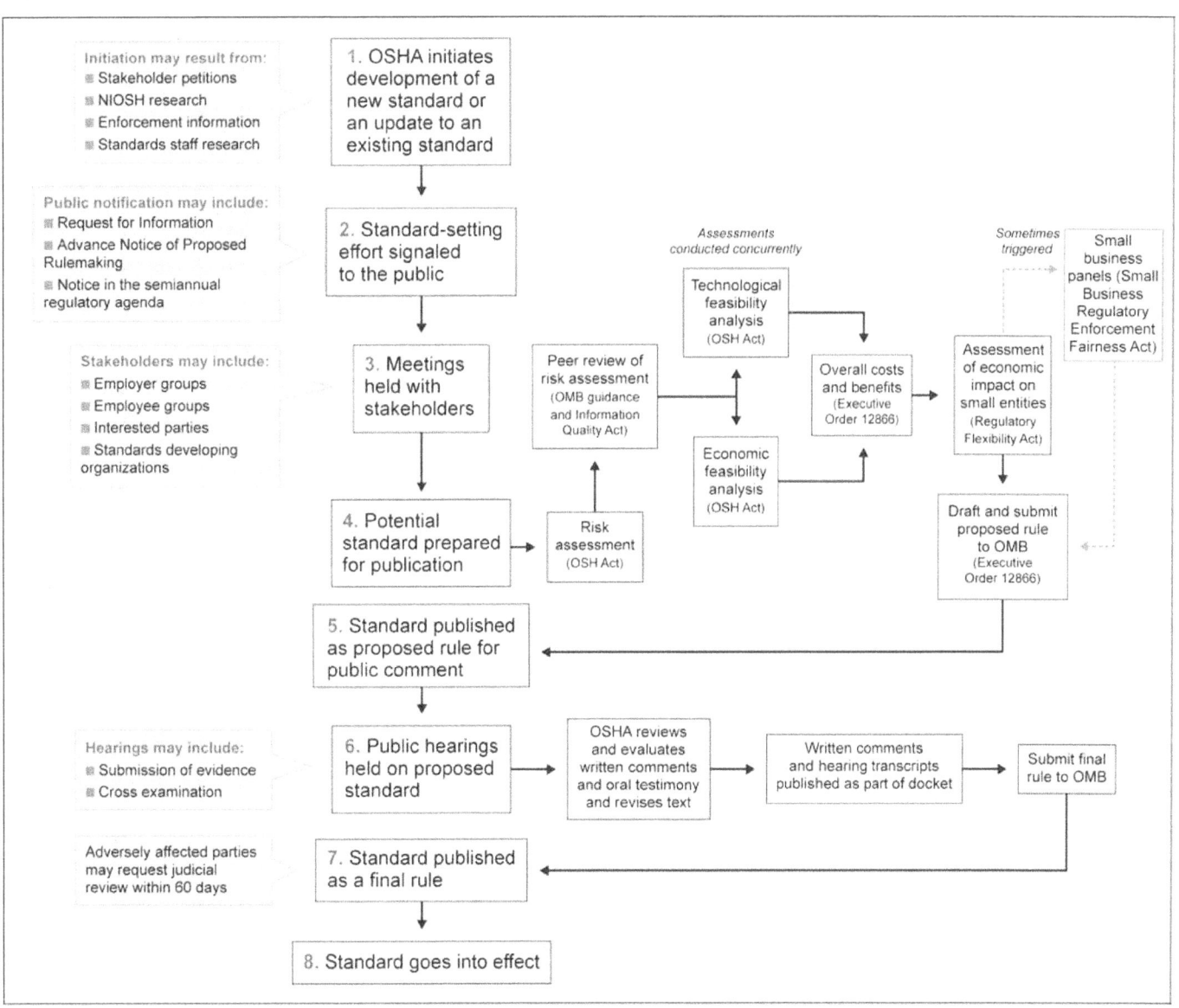

Sources: GAO analysis of interviews with agency officials and relevant federal laws and regulations

Note: This figure is for illustrative purposes only. Not all steps identified here may be performed for all standards and some standards may involve additional steps not included here.

The process for developing OSHA standards varies, but the typical process involves multiple steps. After OSHA initiates a standard-setting effort, staff typically schedule meetings with stakeholders—employer groups, worker groups, and other interested parties—to solicit feedback and discuss issues related to the potential standard, including its potential cost to employers.[25]

Concurrently with these meetings, OSHA staff and contractors perform technological and economic feasibility analyses using data gathered by visiting worksites in industries that will be affected by the potential standard. These analyses are necessary because the Supreme Court has held that the OSH Act requires that standards be both technologically and economically feasible.[26] In addition, courts have held that OSHA must evaluate economic and technological feasibility on an industry-by-industry basis,[27] which requires that the agency research all applications of the hazard being regulated, as well as the expected cost for mitigating exposure to that hazard, in every industry. For the technological feasibility analysis, staff identify the controls required by the standard and determine if each of them is technologically feasible for employers to implement. Agency officials told us this is an enormous undertaking because, for example, sometimes there are no sources of information on the applications of various chemicals or technologies. According to OSHA officials, this also requires visits to multiple worksites, and because these visits are generally conducted on a voluntary basis rather than under OSHA's inspection authority, OSHA staff or its contractors can only visit worksites where the employer allows the visit.[28] Collaboration with NIOSH has, at times, helped facilitate these site visits. For example, OSHA officials told us that their staff worked closely with NIOSH staff in developing the technological feasibility analyses or risk assessments for

[25]We use the term "potential standard" to indicate that the development of a standard is in the early stages, and the term "proposed standard" once an agency issues a Notice of Proposed Rulemaking in the *Federal Register*.

[26]*Am. Textile Mfrs. Inst. v. Donovan*, 452 U.S. 490, 513 n.31 (1981).

[27]See *United Steelworkers v. Marshall*, 647 F.2d 1189, 1301 (D.C. Cir. 1980), quoted in *AFL-CIO v. OSHA*, 965 F.2d 962, 980 (11th Cir. 1992).

[28]Labor officials told us that OSHA prefers to conduct these visits on a voluntary basis to encourage employers to provide information about potential hazards and controls, since employers tend to be less forthcoming with information during an inspection for enforcement purposes.

standards on butadiene, methylene chloride, hexavalent chromium, silica, and diacetyl. When OSHA performs the economic feasibility analysis, it concludes that a standard is economically feasible if the affected industry or industries will maintain long-term profitability and competitiveness.[29] To do this, staff and contractors, by analyzing information they collect when visiting worksites, must assess the extent to which employers in the affected industries can afford to implement the required controls. In addition to the site visits, OSHA staff sometimes conducts industry-wide surveys to determine baseline practices and collect other relevant information needed for the technological and economic feasibility analyses. According to OSHA officials, the process of developing a survey and having it approved by OMB takes a minimum of 1 year.[30]

In addition to the feasibility analyses, OSHA staff generally must also conduct economic analyses. First, OSHA must assess the costs and benefits of significant standards as required by Executive Order 12866.[31] Second, under the Small Business Regulatory Enforcement Fairness Act of 1996, if OSHA determines that a potential standard would have a significant economic impact on a substantial number of small entities, such as businesses, it is one of three federal agencies that must initiate a panel process that seeks and considers input from representatives of the affected small businesses.[32] The small business panel process takes several months of work that many other federal regulatory agencies do not have to complete in order to issue regulations. Agency officials told us they want to consult with small businesses, but that the provisions laid out

---

[29]The Supreme Court has held this approach to be reasonable under the OSH Act. *Am. Textile Mfrs. Inst. v. Donovan*, 452 U.S. 490, 531 n.55 (1981).

[30]Under the Paperwork Reduction Act of 1980, as amended, federal agencies may not conduct or sponsor the collection of information from 10 or more persons without first allowing an opportunity for public comment and obtaining OMB approval. 44 U.S.C. §§ 3502, 3507.

[31]Executive Order 12866 requires that OSHA provide an assessment of the potential overall costs and benefits for significant rules to OMB. For rules that are "economically significant," the agency must also submit a more detailed cost-benefit analysis. Economically significant rules are those that will have an annual effect on the economy of $100 million or more or will adversely affect in a material way the economy, a sector of the economy, productivity, competition, jobs, the environment, public health or safety, or state, local, or tribal governments or communities. See 58 Fed. Reg. 51,735 (Sept. 30, 1993).

[32]5 U.S.C. § 609(b), (d). OSHA staff must work with the Small Business Administration to set up the small business panels. The other two agencies that are subject to this requirement are EPA and the Consumer Financial Protection Bureau.

in the requirement make it too formal a process and are duplicative of the public hearings they hold after publishing the proposed rule. Finally, according to OMB guidelines, if a potential standard is projected to have an economic impact of more than $500 million, OSHA must initiate a peer review of the underlying scientific analyses.[33]

After completing the above steps, OSHA submits the preamble and text of the potential standard to OMB for review.[34] OSHA then publishes a Notice of Proposed Rulemaking in the *Federal Register* to alert the public that OSHA intends to issue a new final standard and to invite interested parties to comment on the proposed standard. Although OSHA is only required under the OSH Act hold public hearings upon request, as a general practice, officials told us that OSHA holds such hearings and has issued regulations governing its hearing procedures.[35] Notably, an administrative law judge presides over the hearings, and stakeholders have the opportunity to submit evidence to support their views on specific provisions of the proposed standards. The administrative law judge may also permit cross-examination by stakeholders or OSHA attorneys to bolster or challenge testimony presented during the hearing. Finally, stakeholders can submit data and other written documents subsequent to the hearing that OSHA must consider when crafting the final standard.

GAO has reported that, while regulatory agencies are generally subject to a number of rulemaking requirements, many rules do not trigger certain requirements.[36] In OSHA's case, for example, if the agency certifies that a standard would *not* have a significant economic impact on a substantial number of small entities, OSHA would not be required to conduct small

---

[33]Information Quality Bulletin for Peer Review, 70 Fed. Reg. 2664 (Jan. 14, 2005). A peer review is also required for scientific assessments determined to be novel, controversial, or precedent-setting or have significant interagency interest.

[34]Executive Order 12866 requires that OMB review all significant regulatory actions prior to their publication in the *Federal Register*. The executive order generally limits this review period to a maximum of 90 days; however, this period may be extended on a one-time basis for up to 30 days upon written approval of the OMB Director, or indefinitely at the request of the head of the rulemaking agency.

[35]See 29 C.F.R. §§ 1911.15 through 1911.18.

[36]GAO, *Federal Rulemaking: Improvements Needed to Monitoring and Evaluation of Rules Development as Well as to the Transparency of OMB Regulatory Reviews*, GAO-09-205 (Washington, D.C.: Apr. 20, 2009).

GAO-12-330 Workplace Safety and Health

business panels, which agency officials estimated adds about 8 months to the standard-setting process.

Shifting Priorities

According to agency officials and experts, OSHA's priorities may change as a result of changes within OSHA, Labor, Congress, or the presidential administration. During the 30-year period covered by our review, administrations have alternately favored and resisted the development of new federal regulations or revisions of existing regulations. For example, officials told us that Assistant Secretaries typically serve for about 3 years, and that new appointees tend to change the agency's priorities. Some agency officials and experts told us that, regardless of the agency leadership's motivation for changes in priority, these changes often cause delays in the process of setting standards. Further, officials told us that, ultimately, political appointees make decisions about what standards, if any, to pursue based on their goals and the agency's resources.

Other experts described instances in which changes in the agency's standard-setting priorities affected the process. One example some cited was OSHA's efforts to develop the ergonomics standard. OSHA worked for several years in the 1990s to develop a proposed rule on ergonomics to address workers' exposure to risk factors leading to musculoskeletal disorders. After being in the preproposal stage through much of the 1990s, there was interest in the late 1990s for OSHA to publish a proposed rule, and OSHA issued a final standard just 1 year after publishing the proposed rule.[37] Several experts and agency officials noted that, in order to develop the rule so quickly, the vast majority of OSHA's standard-setting resources were focused on this rulemaking effort, taking attention away from several standards that previously had been a priority. Agency officials told us, for example, that work on this standard used nearly 50 full-time staff in OSHA's standards office, half the staff

---

[37]See 65 Fed. Reg. 68,262 (Nov. 14, 2000).

economists, and 7 or 8 attorneys, compared with the more typical 5 total staff assigned to develop a new standard.[38]

Standard of Judicial Review

The standard of judicial review that applies to OSHA standards if they are challenged in court also affects OSHA's time frames because it requires more robust research and analysis, according to some experts and agency officials. OSHA standards are subject to a different standard of judicial review than most other federal regulatory agencies' regulations. Instead of the arbitrary and capricious test provided for under the APA, the OSH Act directs courts to review OSHA's standards using a more stringent legal standard: it provides that a standard shall be upheld if supported by "substantial evidence in the record considered as a whole."[39] According to some experts and agency officials, this more stringent standard requires a higher level of scrutiny by the courts and, therefore, requires OSHA staff to perform more extensive research and analysis to support a new standard. For example, OSHA officials explained that the substantial evidence standard requires that OSHA staff conduct a large volume of detailed research in order to understand all industrial processes that involve the hazard being regulated and to ensure that a given hazard control would be feasible for each process.

Data Challenges and Response to Past Adverse Court Decisions

OSHA officials and experts discussed two additional factors that cause OSHA officials to perform an extensive amount of work in developing standards, which are related to the factors described above.

Substantial Data Challenges

Agency officials said that a dearth of available scientific data for some hazards; having to review and evaluate scientific studies; and limited access to worksites to collect information required to demonstrate the

---

[38]After OSHA issued the ergonomics standard, it was met with substantial opposition within Congress and, 4 months after it was issued, the standard was invalidated in accordance with the Congressional Review Act. Under the Congressional Review Act, if Congress enacts a joint resolution of disapproval within a certain time period after a rule is submitted to Congress, the rule shall not take effect (or shall not continue in effect) and it may not be reissued in substantially the same form unless expressly authorized by subsequent law. For a rule to be invalidated, the President must sign the joint resolution of disapproval, or, if vetoed by the President, Congress must override that veto. 5 U.S.C. §§ 801-802. A joint resolution disapproving the ergonomics rule was enacted on March 20, 2001. Pub. L. No. 107-5, 115 Stat. 7 (2001).

[39]29 U.S.C. § 655(f).

need for or feasibility of a standard contribute to substantial challenges to attaining information required for setting standards. They cited court decisions interpreting the OSH Act's requirements as one of the reasons they must rigorously support the need for and feasibility of standards. For example, in 1980, the Supreme Court held that before it can issue a standard, OSHA must determine that the standard is necessary to remedy a "significant risk" of material health impairment among workers.[40] As a result of this decision, OSHA generally conducts quantitative risk assessments for each health standard, which it must ensure are supported by substantial evidence.[41] According to agency officials, this decision essentially established a standard of medical and scientific certainty and has resulted in OSHA staff having to spend an inordinate amount of effort gathering data to support the need for a standard.

Response to Adverse Court Decisions

OSHA's standard-setting process has been significantly influenced by court decisions interpreting statutory requirements. A key example is the 1980 "benzene decision," in which the Supreme Court invalidated an OSHA standard that set a new exposure limit for benzene because OSHA failed to make a determination that benzene posed a "significant risk" of material health impairment under workplace conditions permitted by the current standard.[42] Another example is a 1992 decision in which the U.S. Court of Appeals for the Eleventh Circuit struck down an OSHA health standard that would have set or updated the permissible exposure limit (PEL) for over 400 air contaminants.[43] In that case, the court found that OSHA had not adequately demonstrated that current exposure to each hazard posed significant risk, or that each standard reduced that risk to

---

[40] *Indus. Union Dep't, AFL-CIO v. Am. Petroleum Inst.*, 448 U.S. 607, 639 (1980).

[41] Although the decision interpreted a provision of the OSH Act that applied only to health hazards, Labor officials said that there is little practical distinction between the evidence OSHA must compile to support health standards compared to safety standards. According to OSHA's approach to setting safety standards, which has been upheld by the U.S. Court of Appeals for the D.C. Circuit, a safety standard must provide a "high degree of worker protection"—a showing that differs only "modestly" from that required for health standards. See *UAW v. OSHA*, 37 F.3d 665, 669 (D.C. Cir. 1994).

[42] *Indus. Union Dep't, AFL-CIO v. Am. Petroleum Inst.*, 448 U.S. 607, 639 (1980).

[43] *AFL-CIO v. OSHA*, 965 F.2d 962, 986-87 (11th Cir. 1992). A PEL refers to the limit on the amount or concentration of a hazardous substance in the air or to which skin is exposed.

the extent feasible. Labor officials told us that the court's decision discouraged them from trying to expedite the standard-setting process by combining many standards into one rulemaking effort.[44] Several experts with whom we spoke observed that such adverse court decisions have contributed to an institutional culture of trying to make OSHA standards impervious to future adverse decisions. These experts cited the threat of litigation as a disincentive to issuing standards. In contrast, agency officials commented that while OSHA tries to avoid lawsuits that might ultimately invalidate a standard, in general OSHA does not try to make a standard "bulletproof." Agency officials noted the agency is frequently sued.

OSHA has Authority to Address Urgent Hazards through Emergency Temporary Standards, Enforcement, and Education

Although It Has the Authority, OSHA Has Found it Difficult to Issue Emergency Temporary Standards

OSHA has not issued any emergency temporary standards in nearly 30 years, citing, among other reasons, legal and logistical challenges. Section 6(c) of the OSH Act authorizes OSHA to issue these standards without following the typical standard-setting process if two legal requirements are met. The Secretary of Labor must determine that: (1) workers are exposed to grave danger from exposure to substances or agents determined to be toxic or physically harmful, or from new hazards, and (2) an emergency temporary standard is necessary to protect workers from that danger.[45] An emergency temporary standard becomes effective immediately upon publication in the *Federal Register* and must

---

[44]The court's decision did not prohibit OSHA from setting standards for multiple hazards in a single rulemaking, rather it clarified that the agency must make the required findings under the OSH Act, supported by substantial evidence, for each standard.

[45]Codified at 29 U.S.C. § 655(c).

be replaced within 6 months by a permanent standard issued using the process specified in section 6(b). OSHA officials told us that meeting the statutory requirements and issuing a permanent standard within the 6-month time frame has proven difficult. Furthermore, OSHA's emergency temporary standards have received close scrutiny by federal courts, whose decisions have characterized OSHA's emergency temporary standard authority as an extraordinary power to be used only in limited situations.[46]

Legal Challenges

OSHA officials noted that the emergency temporary standard authority remains available, but the legal requirements to issue such a standard are difficult to meet. OSHA issued nine emergency temporary standards between 1971, when the agency was established, and 1983, and none since that year. Five of those nine emergency temporary standards were either stayed or invalidated, at least in part, by federal courts.[47]

For OSHA to satisfy the first of the OSH Act's two requirements for issuing an emergency temporary standard, the agency must determine that workers will be exposed to grave danger during the time an emergency temporary standard is in effect. Establishing sufficient evidence of grave danger to withstand a court challenge can be difficult, even for substances whose hazards are well-known, such as asbestos. In 1983, OSHA issued an emergency temporary standard lowering the PEL for asbestos, which was subsequently challenged in federal court by representatives of the asbestos industry. The court held that OSHA failed to show sufficient evidence that workers faced grave danger from exposure under current limits for the 6 months the emergency temporary standard would be in effect.[48] OSHA had estimated, based on

---

[46]See, for example, *Public Citizen Health Research Group v. Auchter*, 702 F.2d 1150, 1155 (D.C. Cir. 1983), quoted in *Asbestos Info. Ass'n v. OSHA*, 727 F.2d 415, 422 (5th Cir. 1984).

[47]A stay means the court issued an order postponing the emergency temporary standard from going into effect. See *Asbestos Info. Ass'n v. OSHA*, 727 F.2d 415 (5th Cir. 1984), *Taylor Diving & Salvage Co. v. U.S. Dep't. of Labor*, 537 F.2d 819 (5th Cir.1976), *Florida Peach Growers Ass'n v. U.S. Dep't. of Labor*, 489 F.2d 120 (5th Cir. 1974), and *Dry Color Mfrs. Ass'n v. Brennan*, 486 F.2d 98 (3d Cir.1973). An emergency temporary standard on benzene was stayed in an unpublished decision by the U.S. Court of Appeals for the Fifth Circuit. See *Indus. Union Dep't, AFL-CIO v. Am. Petroleum Inst.*, 448 U.S. 607, 623 (1980).

[48]*Asbestos Info. Ass'n v. OSHA*, 727 F.2d 415, 425-27 (5th Cir. 1984).

mathematical projections from long-term epidemiological studies, that during the 6 months the emergency temporary standard would be in effect, it could prevent at least 80 eventual asbestos-related deaths. However, the court found these projections too uncertain to establish a grave risk over a 6-month period and noted that the type of analysis OSHA used merited the public scrutiny of the notice and comment standard-setting process.

OSHA has also found it challenging to meet the second OSH Act requirement: establishing that an emergency temporary standard is necessary to protect workers from the grave danger. In the asbestos case, the court found that OSHA was on its way to issuing a permanent standard within a year, already had the authority to conduct the education activities the emergency temporary standard contained, and could achieve many of the same benefits by increasing enforcement of the existing standard. The court, therefore, invalidated the emergency temporary asbestos standard because OSHA failed to meet both of the OSH Act's requirements. OSHA officials cited diacetyl, a food flavoring ingredient, as a recent example of a hazardous substance for which the OSH Act's second requirement might have been difficult to meet if the agency had chosen to pursue an emergency temporary standard. In 2006, the agency was urged to issue an emergency temporary standard for diacetyl after investigations showed its association with severe, irreversible lung disease among workers in microwave popcorn factories. OSHA officials told us they could likely have established that diacetyl exposure under then-current workplace conditions presented grave danger to workers in the near term. These officials noted, however, that because manufacturers responded quickly after diacetyl's danger became clear, OSHA had less evidence that an emergency temporary standard was necessary. For example, they noted that manufacturers responded with a combination of measures including improved ventilation and housekeeping, reducing the concentration of diacetyl used, and substituting other ingredients.

Logistical Challenge

In addition to the legal requirements, OSHA has found that issuing an emergency temporary standard presents a logistical challenge. OSHA's emergency temporary standards are effective on the date of publication in the *Federal Register*, but they must be replaced within 6 months by a permanent standard.[49] This means OSHA must compile the same evidence required for the typical standard-setting process—which, as noted above, involves engaging with stakeholders and can take many years—in this abbreviated time frame. OSHA officials noted that the Congress intended this emergency temporary standard-setting authority to be used under very limited circumstances.

OSHA has not issued an emergency temporary standard since 1983, despite many requests that it do so. Labor unions and public health and other advocacy organizations continue to petition OSHA to issue emergency temporary standards to address a variety of workplace hazards. According to OSHA records, it has received 23 petitions to issue emergency temporary standards on hazardous chemicals, such as formaldehyde, and also for safety hazards such as shock or injury from unsecured equipment. One petition, submitted in September 2011, urges OSHA to issue an emergency temporary standard to protect workers from potentially fatal exposure to heat. Although OSHA has generally denied these petitions, officials told us the agency considers whether to issue an emergency temporary standard and takes the information into account when setting its priorities for permanent standards.

OSHA Addresses Urgent Hazards through Enforcement and Education

OSHA uses enforcement and education as alternatives to issuing emergency temporary standards to respond relatively quickly to urgent workplace hazards. OSHA officials consider their enforcement and education activities complementary: a high-profile citation or enforcement initiative on an urgent hazard generates attention that can improve worker safety industry-wide.

Enforcement

OSHA may cite employers for failing to adequately protect workers from a specific workplace hazard even if it has not set a standard on that hazard. Under section 5(a)(1) of the OSH Act, known as the general duty clause, OSHA has the authority to issue citations to employers even in the absence of a specific standard under certain circumstances. The general duty clause requires employers to provide a workplace free from recognized hazards that are causing, or are likely to cause, death or

---

[49]The emergency temporary standard serves as the proposed rule for a permanent standard to be issued within 6 months, in accordance with all the procedural requirements for OSHA's standard setting under section 6(b) of the OSH Act.

serious physical harm to their employees.[50] OSHA relied on the general duty clause when it cited Walmart for inadequate crowd management in the 2008 trampling death of a worker. OSHA's investigation found that the company failed to protect its employees from the known risks of being crushed or suffocated by a large unmanaged crowd—in this case, about 2,000 shoppers surging into the store for a holiday sale. To cite an employer under the general duty clause, OSHA officials told us they must, among other things, have evidence that the hazard is "recognized" in the industry and that the employer failed to take reasonable protective measures. According to OSHA officials, using the general duty clause requires significant agency resources so is not always a viable option, for example when OSHA cannot prove an employer knows the hazard exists or when a hazard is just emerging.

Some of OSHA's standards require general protective measures that are sufficiently broad to cover a variety of hazardous substances or practices. Such standards may be the basis for enforcement actions regarding urgent hazards that are not the subject of a specific standard. OSHA officials explained that not every conceivable workplace hazard can be the subject of its own standard. The agency has issued specific exposure limits for some hazardous substances, such as formaldehyde, but indicated it would be impossible to test and establish specific exposure limits for all chemicals present in the modern workplace. OSHA's general standards include, among others, requirements for employers to follow protective housekeeping practices, provide respiratory protection under certain conditions, and inform workers about hazardous chemicals they are exposed to on the job.[51]

Education

OSHA uses education to promote voluntary protective measures against urgent hazards along with its enforcement and standard-setting activities. Standards and enforcement are critical parts of OSHA's education activities: standards inform employers about their responsibilities, and enforcement initiatives raise awareness of urgent hazards. OSHA officials believe high-profile citations serve to focus attention throughout the relevant industry and can create a ripple effect of improved worker protection. In addition to setting standards, OSHA offers on-site

---

[50]Codified at 29 U.S.C. § 654(a)(1).

[51]See, for example, 29 C.F.R. §§ 1910.22(a) (housekeeping), 1910.134 (respiratory protection), and 1910.1200 (hazard communication).

consultations and publishes health and safety information to inform employers and workers about urgent hazards. If its inspectors discover a particular hazard, OSHA may send letters to all employers where the hazard is likely to be present to inform them about the hazard and their responsibility to protect their employees.

OSHA officials also use education to improve safety in the near term while the agency compiles the information necessary to develop a standard. For example, OSHA decided not to issue an emergency temporary standard on diacetyl in part because, as it gathered evidence to support the standard, employers implemented changes to improve worker safety. As evidence mounts that other ingredients in food flavorings may be hazardous, OSHA is gathering information but has not yet published a proposed standard on diacetyl. OSHA has, in the meantime, published educational documents such as alerts and information bulletins for employers on diacetyl and flavorings in general, describing protective measures, compliance assistance programs, and employer responsibilities under the OSH Act and existing OSHA standards.[52] The agency has also developed material for workers, giving them the information they need to determine when they may be exposed to diacetyl or similar substances and the types of protection they need.

OSHA's education efforts also address other hazards for which it has received petitions to issue emergency temporary standards. For example, OSHA officials told us they are addressing the risks of exposure to heat primarily through education, along with targeted enforcement in cases where workers are known to be most at risk. OSHA's education efforts on this hazard include an initiative intended to reach and educate agricultural workers through training materials designed to be culturally appropriate and accessible, including a train-the-trainer approach for wide distribution. These training materials were supplemented by public service radio announcements intended to reach workers at risk of heat-related illness.

---

[52]OSHA has stated that some of the most relevant applicable standards include those requiring employers to provide respiratory protection, 29 C.F.R. § 1910.134, and inform employees about hazardous chemicals and protective measures, 29 C.F.R. § 1910.1200.

Other Regulatory Agencies' Experiences Offer Limited Insight into OSHA's Challenges

Although the rulemaking experiences of two other federal agencies shed some light on OSHA's challenges, their statutory framework and resources differ too markedly for them to be models for OSHA's standard–setting process. Other regulatory agencies may also face challenges similar to OSHA's. For example, as GAO has previously reported, EPA has faced difficulties regulating under the Toxic Substances Control Act of 1976.[53] Some of these differences in statutory frameworks and resources may facilitate rulemaking efforts at other agencies. For example, EPA is directed to regulate specified air pollutants and review its existing regulations within specific time frames under section 112 of the Clean Air Act, and MSHA benefits from a narrower scope of authority than OSHA and has more specialized expertise as a result of its more limited jurisdiction.

EPA

Similar to OSHA, EPA's Office of Air and Radiation regulates a wide range of hazards across diverse industries to protect the public health. This office implements the Clean Air Act, including section 112, which requires EPA to regulate certain sources of air pollution and specifies the substances to be controlled.[54] For example, under section 112, EPA must establish standards for sources of 187 specific hazardous air pollutants.[55] EPA officials told us that this provision gave the agency clear requirements and statutory deadlines for regulating hazardous air

---

[53]See GAO, *Chemical Regulation: Observations on Improving the Toxic Substances Control Act,* GAO-10-292T (Washington, D.C.: Dec. 2, 2009); and GAO, *Chemical Regulation: Options Exist to Improve EPA's Ability to Assess Health Risks and Manage Its Chemical Review Program,* GAO-05-458 (Washington, D.C.: June 13, 2005). For this review, we initially included EPA's efforts under section 6 of this act; however, we concluded that these efforts did not offer insights for OSHA because of the office's limited recent standard-setting experience. For more information on our methodology, see appendix I.

[54]42 U.S.C. § 7412. Section 112 of the Clean Air Act specifies a list of hazardous air pollutants whose emissions are to be controlled under its provisions. After identifying the pollutants to be regulated, the statute directs EPA to impose technology-based standards on industry to reduce emissions. As a second step, within 8 years of issuance of the initial technology-based standards, EPA is to review the remaining risks to the public and issue health-based standards if necessary to provide an ample margin of safety to protect public health or to prevent an adverse environmental effect. Finally, the Clean Air Act requires that EPA review and, if necessary, revise the technology-based standards at least every 8 years, taking into account developments in practices, processes, and control technologies.

[55]The provision also authorizes EPA to, by rule, add or remove pollutants from the list on the basis of specified findings.

pollutants, which it previously lacked.[56] In contrast, some experts and agency officials we spoke with identified OSHA's relatively broad discretion to set and change its regulatory agenda as a contributing factor to the length of time it takes OSHA to issue standards. Even with this relatively specific statutory mandate, EPA has faced challenges implementing its section 112 mandate, such as insufficient funding and court-imposed deadlines that make it difficult for the agency itself to implement its own agenda.[57]

EPA also has a statutory mandate to periodically review the standards issued under section 112. For example, section 112 requires that EPA set technology-based standards for stationary sources of hazardous air pollutants, and further requires that EPA review these standards at least every 8 years and revise them, as necessary, taking into account developments in practices, processes, and control technologies.[58] In contrast, the OSH Act does not specify when OSHA is to revise its standards. OSHA's attempt to update its standards efficiently—by lowering the PELs for 212 air contaminants in one rulemaking—was struck down by a federal court.[59] The court held that OSHA failed to show adequate evidence that each individual substance presented a significant risk at the existing exposure limit, or that the lower limit would reduce the risk to workers to the extent feasible. OSHA and Labor officials noted that, because the agency lacks an efficient update process, many of its standards lag behind advances in technology.

Section 112 of the Clean Air Act requires EPA to set technology-based standards for sources of listed hazardous air pollutants. In setting these standards, EPA does not have to establish evidence of a listed pollutant's

---

[56]However, as GAO reported in 2006, EPA failed to meet some of its statutory deadlines under section 112 of the Clean Air Act. See GAO, *Clean Air Act: EPA Should Improve the Management of its Air Toxics Program,* GAO 06-669 (Washington, D.C.: June 23, 2006).

[57]GAO-06-669.

[58]42 U.S.C. § 7412(d)(6).

[59]*AFL-CIO v. OSHA,* 965 F.2d 962, 986-87 (11th Cir. 1992). The revision to OSHA's Air Contaminants standard addressed a total of 428 hazardous substances by setting new limits for 164 previously unregulated substances, lowering limits for 212 others, and leaving intact limits for 52 substances OSHA had proposed to change in its Notice of Proposed Rulemaking. In determining the limits, OSHA relied upon limits recommended or adopted by entities such as NIOSH and the American Conference of Governmental Industrial Hygienists. 54 Fed. Reg. 2332, 2333 (Jan. 19, 1989).

risks to human health or the environment.[60] In contrast, OSHA must determine that significant risks to workers are present under current conditions before it can establish or change existing standards. OSHA has had to perform a specific risk assessment for every new toxic agent for which it intends to set a PEL.

MSHA

MSHA's mission is more focused than OSHA's because its authority is limited to one industry and it can target its regulatory resources more easily. In addition, the Federal Mine Safety and Health Act of 1977 requires that MSHA inspect each mine in the United States at least two times a year, which facilitates its regulatory work.[61] Officials at MSHA noted that both this frequent on-site presence and relatively homogenous industry helps agency staff maintain a current knowledge base.[62] MSHA officials contrasted this with the vast array of workplaces and types of industries OSHA oversees. Officials with OSHA and Labor noted that OSHA's scope of authority is so large that it cannot inspect more than a fraction of workplaces in any given year. As a result, OSHA and Labor officials told us they can call upon inspectors when researching a standard but must often supplement the agency's inside knowledge by conducting site visits using OSHA staff or contractors.

MSHA's legal framework may also present fewer challenges to standard setting than OSHA's. First, MSHA standards are subject to the arbitrary and capricious standard of review, unlike OSHA standards, which are reviewed under the generally more stringent substantial evidence standard. Second, according to MSHA officials, the agency has met the statutory requirements for the five emergency temporary standards it has issued since 1987, and no legal challenges to these standards were filed. Similar to OSHA's authority to issue emergency temporary standards, MSHA has statutory authority to issue "an emergency temporary

---

[60]EPA generally must show evidence of such effects in order to add other pollutants to the list. For example, EPA is required to periodically review the list of hazardous air pollutants and add new pollutants to the list upon finding that they present, or may present, a threat of adverse effects on human health or the environment. 42 U.S.C. § 7412(b)(2).

[61]30 U.S.C. § 813(a).

[62]MSHA officials, however, noted that the agency strained its resources in the sustained effort to issue regulations required by the Mine Improvement and New Emergency Response Act of 2006, Pub. L. No. 109-236, 120 Stat. 493, which amended the Federal Mine Safety and Health Act of 1977.

mandatory health or safety standard" without following the APA's notice and comment rulemaking procedures if the Secretary of Labor determines that (1) miners are exposed to grave danger from exposure to substances or agents determined to be toxic or physically harmful, or to other hazards, and (2) such a standard is necessary to protect miners from such danger.[63] MSHA's most recent emergency temporary standard required underground bituminous coal mine operators to increase the incombustible content of rock, coal, and other dust, in order to address the risk of explosion posed by such dust.[64]

Both OSHA and MSHA supplement their employees' knowledge by calling upon the expertise at NIOSH, with MSHA benefiting from a specialized research group within NIOSH focused on the mining industry. According to officials with both NIOSH and OSHA, coordination between the two has varied over time and has improved significantly in recent years. For example, in 2011, NIOSH and OSHA adopted a Memorandum of Understanding that provides OSHA with access to specified NIOSH data on the health hazards of diacetyl and allows OSHA to coordinate with NIOSH in preparing a risk assessment to support the development of a new diacetyl standard.

---

[63]30 U.S.C. § 811(b). After it issues an emergency temporary standard, MSHA has 9 months to issue a permanent standard, compared to the 6 months OSHA has to issue a permanent standard after issuing an emergency temporary standard under the OSH Act.

[64]75 Fed. Reg. 57,849 (Sept. 23, 2010).

Experts Suggested Many Ideas to Improve OSHA's Standard-Setting Process, Including More Interagency Coordination and Statutory Deadlines

Agency officials and occupational safety and health experts shared their understanding of the challenges facing OSHA and offered ideas for improving the agency's standard-setting process. Some of the following ideas for improvement involve substantial procedural changes that may in some cases be beyond the scope of OSHA's authority and require amending existing laws, including the OSH Act. The following ideas represent those most frequently mentioned in our interviews by agency officials and experts:[65]

- Improve coordination with other agencies

- Expand use of voluntary consensus standards

- Impose statutory deadlines

- Adopt a priority-setting process

- Allow alternatives for supporting feasibility

- Change the standard of judicial review

- More frequently use emergency temporary standard authority

- Use of the general duty clause for enforcement

Improve Coordination with Other Federal Agencies to Leverage Expertise

To fully leverage expertise at other federal agencies, experts and agency officials suggest improving interagency coordination. Specifically, they indicated that OSHA has not fully leveraged available expertise at other federal agencies, especially NIOSH, when developing and issuing its standards. As mentioned previously, NIOSH conducts research and makes recommendations on occupational safety and health, and it was created at the same time as OSHA by the OSH Act. OSHA has a number of staff with subject matter expertise relevant to standard setting, including industrial hygienists and scientists, but the agency does not always take advantage of the expertise and data at NIOSH on

---

[65]The last two ideas for OSHA mentioned here—to more frequently use the emergency temporary standard authority and to use the general duty clause for enforcement—are not included in the discussion below because they are addressed in previous sections of this report.

occupational hazards. One expert noted that NIOSH is uniquely positioned as a primary research institution to help OSHA develop standards using EPA-produced data and analysis on chemical hazards. OSHA officials said their agency's staff consider NIOSH's input on an ad hoc basis, but do not routinely work closely with NIOSH staff to analyze risks of occupational hazards. An OSHA official cited one case in which OSHA staff worked closely with NIOSH staff to prepare the technological feasibility analysis for a proposed silica standard, drawing on an extensive body of work on dust control technology by NIOSH engineers. In addition, officials described other cases of collaboration between the two agencies during OSHA's process of visiting worksites. However, NIOSH officials told us that this type of coordination has been more common recently than it was in the past, when the two agencies performed separate risk assessments for hazards, such as hexavalent chromium.

OSHA officials stated that collaborating with NIOSH on risk assessments could reduce the time it takes to develop a standard by several months. OSHA and NIOSH have coordinated on a number of OSHA standards projects; currently, the two agencies have a Memorandum of Understanding stipulating that NIOSH will perform the risk assessment for the OSHA standard on diacetyl. However, some experts and officials at both agencies noted that collaborating in a more systematic way could facilitate OSHA's standard-setting process.

Expand OSHA's Ability to Use Industry Voluntary Consensus Standards

To ensure that OSHA's standards keep pace with changes in technology and best practices, experts suggested the agency be allowed to more easily adopt industry voluntary consensus standards. According to OSHA officials, many OSHA standards incorporate or reference outdated consensus standards, which results in challenges for employers in complying with the standards and OSHA in enforcing them. Officials also said that the majority of OSHA's health standards were adopted from existing federal standards—originally adopted under the Walsh-Healy Act—during the agency's first 2 years using section 6(a) of the OSH Act, which directed OSHA to set standards without following the typical section 6(b) standard-setting procedures or the APA. Although current at the time, many industry consensus standards have since been updated to reflect advancements in technology and science. However, according to OSHA, most of OSHA's standards have not been similarly updated, so employers following current industry consensus standards may be out of compliance with OSHA's standards. As a result, some employers may be discouraged from updating processes or technology at their worksites in order to avoid OSHA citations. One expert said, and OSHA reported, that this could leave workers at these worksites exposed to hazards that are insufficiently addressed by OSHA standards that are based on out-of-date technology or processes. OSHA has reported that these types of standards are challenging because their inspectors must spend time addressing them during worksite inspections. Additionally, officials told us that issuing citations to employers that are following the most up-to-date industry consensus standards reflects poorly on the agency. OSHA has attempted to update some of its standards to incorporate advances in technology and science, but the lengthy standard-setting process presents significant challenges for updating them. In accordance with the requirements in the OSH Act and the National Technology Transfer and Advancement Act,[66] when updating its standards, OSHA considers using voluntary consensus standards. However, OSHA officials told us that, since standards developing organizations typically do not have to meet scientific requirements in developing voluntary standards, OSHA's ability to base its standards on voluntary consensus standards is limited because staff must still perform a full quantitative risk assessment for new standards. Since 2004, OSHA has been engaged in an effort to update several of its standards using industry consensus standards, which officials told us started by first identifying standards that would be well-suited to more streamlined rulemaking approaches, such as issuing a direct final rule.[67] For example, they said they chose to update the standard on personal protective equipment first because they expected employers would be amenable to the update, as changes would be consistent with the current industry consensus standard.

---

[66]29 U.S.C. § 655(b)(8), 15 U.S.C. § 272 note.

[67]The APA's notice and comment rulemaking procedures are not required in certain circumstances, such as when an agency finds, for "good cause," that those procedures are "impracticable, unnecessary, or contrary to the public interest." 5 U.S.C. § 553(b). A direct final rule is one alternative rulemaking procedure used by agencies in which the agency publishes a rule in the *Federal Register* with a statement that the rule will be effective on a particular date unless an adverse comment is received within a specified period of time (e.g., 30 days). If an adverse comment is filed, the direct final rule is withdrawn, and the agency may publish the rule as a proposed rule. OSHA's regulations provide that "minor rules or amendments in which the public is not particularly interested" may be issued without the notice and public procedure that would otherwise be required. 29 C.F.R. § 1911.5. According to agency officials, OSHA uses the direct final rule process for noncontroversial rules, but it is unlikely the agency would be able to use it more often in standard setting because of the limited opportunity for public comment.

To address the problem of standards based on outdated consensus standards, experts suggested that Congress pass new legislation that would allow OSHA, through a single rulemaking effort, to revise standards for a group of health hazards based on current industry voluntary consensus standards or the Threshold Limit Values developed by the American Conference of Governmental Industrial Hygienists.[68] In 1989, OSHA attempted to revise the PELs for over 200 air contaminants by combining them into a single rulemaking effort, but the rule was invalidated by the court for failing to follow the OSH Act requirements for each hazard. To save OSHA time, experts specified that any new law to this effect should contain a provision similar to the one in the OSH Act that excused the agency during its first 2 years from following the standard-setting provisions of section 6(b) of the OSH Act or the APA.[69] One potential disadvantage of this proposal is that OSHA may need to do a substantial amount of independent scientific research to ensure that consensus standards are based on sufficient scientific evidence. While such a law, if enacted, could exempt OSHA from conducting this research, an abbreviated regulatory process could also result in standards that fail to reflect relevant stakeholder concerns, such as an imposition of unnecessarily burdensome requirements on employers. For example, one expert stated that, while following the APA process takes time for regulatory agencies, it leads to higher quality standards and ensures that the basis for agency action is clear and defensible. Also, while this change could help ensure that existing OSHA standards are kept up to date, it could divert resources away from efforts to set new standards.

---

[68]This private, not-for-profit, nongovernmental corporation is a scientific association that has developed Threshold Limit Values as guidelines to assist in the control of potential workplace health hazards. In developing these guidelines, committees of experts in public health and related sciences review peer-reviewed scientific literature to determine levels of exposure that the typical worker can experience without adverse health effects. However, the committees consider neither economic nor technological feasibility when determining Threshold Limit Values, nor do they result from a consensus process of agreement among interested stakeholders.

[69]29 U.S.C. § 655(a).

Impose Statutory Deadlines and Provide Relief from Procedural Requirements for Setting Standards

To minimize the time it takes OSHA to develop and issue safety or health standards, experts and agency officials suggested that statutory deadlines for issuing occupational safety and health standards be imposed by Congress and enforced by the courts. OSHA officials indicated that it can be difficult to prioritize standards due to the agency's numerous and sometimes competing goals. In the past, having a statutory deadline, combined with relief from procedural requirements, resulted in OSHA issuing standards more quickly. For example, the Needlestick Safety and Prevention Act directed OSHA to make specified revisions to its bloodborne pathogens standard within 6 months and exempted the agency from the typical procedural requirements under section 6(b) of the OSH Act or the APA.[70] OSHA had already spent some time developing the standard before the law was passed, so it was able to complete the revised standard within the required time frame. Including the time spent on developing the standard before passage of the Act, OSHA completed the revised standard in less than 3 years. Another alternative to the full rulemaking process is for an agency to issue an interim final rule, which is immediately effective as a final rule but still allows for subsequent public comment.[71] However, similar to one of the disadvantages described above, some legal scholars have noted that curtailing the current rulemaking process required by the APA may result in fewer opportunities for public input and possibly decrease the quality of the standard.[72] Also, officials from MSHA told us that statutory deadlines make its priorities clear, but this is sometimes to the detriment of other issues that must be set aside in the meantime. Although a more streamlined approach could reduce opportunities for stakeholder comments and minimize agency flexibility, OSHA has used alternative

---

[70]Pub. L. No. 106-430, 114 Stat. 1901 (2000).

[71]Interim final rules are another alternative to APA notice and comment rulemaking, in addition to direct final rules. In interim final rulemaking, if the public comments persuade the agency that changes are needed in the interim final rule, the agency may revise the rule by publishing a final rule reflecting those changes. Labor officials told us that OSHA generally needs specific statutory authority to set substantive standards using an interim final rule. For example, the Housing and Community Development Act of 1992 required the Secretary of Labor to issue an interim final rule on occupational exposure to lead in the construction industry, to be effective until replaced by a permanent standard. Pub. L. No. 102-550, § 1031, 106 Stat. 3672, 3924.

[72]See, for example, Jacob E. Gersen and Anne Joseph O'Connell, "Deadlines in Administrative Law," *University of Pennsylvania Law Review*, vol. 156 (2007-2008).

rulemaking procedures in the past to issue standards for which officials perceive broad industry support.

Change the Standard of Judicial Review for OSHA Standards

Experts and agency officials suggested OSHA's substantial evidence standard of judicial review be replaced with the arbitrary and capricious standard, which would be more consistent with other federal regulatory agencies. As the court stated in the case involving PELs for 428 air contaminants, under the substantial evidence test, "[the court] must take a 'harder look' at OSHA's action than we would if we were reviewing the action under the more deferential arbitrary and capricious standard applicable to agencies governed by the Administrative Procedure Act."[73] As a result, OSHA officials said they spend a significant amount of time collecting evidence to ensure that its standards can withstand challenge under the substantial evidence standard of judicial review and to satisfy procedural requirements for setting standards. One expert said he understood that OSHA's more stringent standard of judicial review was paired with informal rulemaking procedures as a congressional compromise.

According to the author of a 1999 law review article, one justification for judicial review of agency rulemaking is when there is a genuine concern about the power many agencies have in the regulatory process.[74] If Congress has similar concerns about OSHA, it may be preferable to keep the current standard of review. However, the Administrative Conference of the United States has recommended that Congress amend laws that mandate use of the substantial evidence standard because it can be unnecessarily burdensome for the agency or confusing because it has been inconsistently applied by the courts.[75] As a result, changing the designation for the standard of judicial review to "arbitrary and capricious" could reduce the agency's evidentiary burden.

---

[73]*AFL-CIO v. OSHA*, 965 F.2d 962, 970 (11th Cir. 1992), quoting *Asbestos Info. Ass'n v. OSHA*, 727 F.2d 415, 421 (5th Cir. 1984).

[74]Mark Seidenfeld, "Bending the Rules: Flexible Regulation and Constraints on Agency Discretion," *Administrative Law Review* (spring, 1999).

[75]59 Fed. Reg. 4669, 4670-71 (Feb. 1, 1994). The Administrative Conference of the United States is an independent federal agency that makes recommendations for improving federal agency procedures, including the federal rulemaking process.

Improve Strategies for Supporting Economic and Technological Feasibility Analyses

Experts suggested that OSHA minimize on-site visits by using surveys or basing its analyses on industry best practices, which could reduce the time, expense, and need for industry cooperation in conducting economic and technological feasibility studies. Primarily because OSHA has broad authority to regulate occupational hazards in nearly all private industries, the technological and economic feasibility analyses required by the OSH Act entail an extensive amount of time and resources. OSHA must conduct its feasibility analyses on an industry-by-industry basis, which requires numerous site visits—an activity that is time-consuming and largely dependent on industry cooperation. According to agency officials, in many cases, OSHA hires contractors to gather information from worksites that will support standards' feasibility analyses.

Two experts suggested OSHA could streamline its economic and technological feasibility analyses by surveying worksites rather than visiting them. However, one limitation to this method is that, according to OSHA officials, in-person site visits are imperative for gathering sufficient data in support of most health standards. Specifically, officials told us that to fully understand the industrial processes and application of a chemical to be regulated, OSHA staff or contractors must be able to observe the work being performed and ask questions of workers at the site. In addition, the only way for OSHA to know about ambient chemical levels is to collect on-site air samples all day long. In light of this limitation, this method may be more appropriate for safety hazards. The other method experts suggested is allowing OSHA to base economic and technological feasibility assessments on industry best practices, which one expert noted would require a statutory change. For example, OSHA could base these analyses on the fact that a minimum percentage of workplaces in a particular industry use technology or methods that decrease exposure to hazards. However, the broad scope of OSHA's authority would still result in this being a substantial amount of work at the outset, as OSHA would still be required to determine feasibility on an industry-by-industry basis.

Adopt a Priority-Setting Process for Addressing Hazards

Experts suggested that OSHA develop a priority-setting process for addressing hazards. GAO has reported that, by developing strategies such as aligning agencywide objectives, federal agencies can demonstrate a commitment to a course of action.[76] Similarly, having a

---

[76]GAO, *Managing for Results: Enhancing Agency Use of Performance Information for Management Decision Making,* GAO-05-927 (Washington D.C.: Sept. 9, 2005).

priority-setting process could lead to improved program results. Currently, however, OSHA has no process or guidance to use in setting priorities, as officials told us they do not have a document that explains how priorities are or should be set. OSHA officials also said that ideas for which hazards to regulate come from a number of sources, including petitions from stakeholders, information from NIOSH, OSHA's enforcement efforts, recommendations from the Chemical Safety Board, and staff research. While staff in OSHA's standards office use this information to make recommendations to Labor's Assistant Secretary for OSHA and the Deputy Secretary on which hazards to regulate, not all of their recommendations make it to the agency's regulatory agenda, which is developed according to agency goals and resources. In addition, according to OSHA officials, decisions about which hazards to regulate guide OSHA standards activity for 6 months, the duration of the biannual regulatory agenda. As a result, the ability of the managers of OSHA's standards office to plan with certainty work beyond this 6-month time frame may be limited.

One expert suggested that OSHA develop a priority-setting process that more directly involves stakeholders with expertise in occupational safety and health in recommending new standards. OSHA attempted such a process in 1994 when it initiated a formal priority planning process. However, the expert said that, after an established committee of experts identified a list of priority hazards, the political climate changed with a new Congress that was generally more critical of the role of executive agencies in developing new standards, and OSHA shifted its focus away from this initiative. Nevertheless, this process allowed OSHA to articulate its highest priorities for addressing occupational hazards. Reestablishing a similar priority-setting process could have several benefits for OSHA, such as improving a sense of transparency among stakeholders and facilitating OSHA management's ability to plan its staffing and budgetary needs. However, adopting such a process may not immediately address OSHA's challenges in expeditiously setting standards because a process like this could take time and would require commitment from agency management.

Conclusions

Setting occupational safety and health standards is one of OSHA's primary methods for ensuring that workers are protected from occupational hazards, but OSHA faces a number of challenges in setting these standards promptly and efficiently. The additional procedural requirements established since 1980 by Congress and various executive orders have increased opportunities for stakeholder input in the regulatory process and required agencies to evaluate and explain the need for regulations, but they have also resulted in a more protracted rulemaking process for OSHA and other regulatory agencies. The process for developing new standards for previously unregulated occupational hazards and new hazards that emerge is a lengthy one and can result in periods when there are insufficient protections for workers. Nevertheless, any streamlining of the current process must guarantee sufficient stakeholder input to ensure that the quality of standards does not suffer. In addition, ideas for changes to the regulatory process must weigh the benefits of addressing hazards more quickly against a potential increase in the regulatory burden to be imposed on the regulated community. Most methods for streamlining that have been suggested by experts and agency officials are largely outside of OSHA's authority because many procedural requirements are established by federal statute or executive order. However, OSHA can coordinate more routinely with NIOSH on risk assessments and other analyses required to support the need for standards, saving OSHA time and expense. NIOSH's and OSHA's current efforts to coordinate on the development of a new standard, which officials and staff from both agencies support, provides a useful template for increased and regular coordination on similar efforts.

Recommendation for Executive Action

To enhance collaboration and streamline the development of OSHA's occupational safety and health standards, we recommend that the Secretary of Labor and the Secretary of the Department of Health and Human Services instruct the Assistant Secretary of Labor for Occupational Safety and Health and the Director of the National Institute for Occupational Safety and Health to develop a more formal means of collaboration between the two agencies. Specifically, the two agencies should establish a more consistent and sustained relationship through a formal agreement, such as a Memorandum of Understanding, allowing OSHA to better leverage NIOSH's capacity as a primary research institution when building the scientific record required for standard setting.

Agency Comments

We provided a draft of this report to the six agencies that assisted us in gathering information: Labor (OSHA and MSHA), Department of Health and Human Services (NIOSH), EPA, U.S. Chemical Safety and Hazard Investigation Board, OMB, and the Department of Commerce (National Institute of Standards and Technology). We received written comments from Labor and the Department of Health and Human Services; both sets of comments are reproduced in appendices III and IV, respectively. Both Labor's Assistant Secretary for OSHA and the Department of Health and

Human Services' Assistant Secretary for Legislation agreed with GAO's recommendation. They also both described the ways in which OSHA and NIOSH currently collaborate, each noting the expected benefits of maintaining collaboration through a formalized agreement. Labor's OSHA and MSHA, EPA, and the Department of Commerce also provided technical comments, which we incorporated in the report as appropriate.

As agreed with your offices, unless you publicly announce the contents of this report earlier, we plan no further distribution until 30 days from the report date. At that time, we will send copies to the appropriate congressional committees and other interested parties. In addition, this report will be available at no charge on the GAO website at http://www.gao.gov.

If you or your staff members have any questions about this report, please contact me at (202) 512-7215 or moranr@gao.gov. Contact points for our Offices of Congressional Relations and Public Affairs may be found on the last page of this report. Key contributors to this report are listed in appendix V.

Revae E. Moran

Revae Moran, Director
Education, Workforce
    and Income Security Issues

List of Committees

The Honorable Tom Harkin
Chairman
Committee on Health, Education, Labor, and Pensions
United States Senate

The Honorable Patty Murray
Chairman
Subcommittee on Employment and Workplace Safety
Committee on Health, Education, Labor, and Pensions
United States Senate

The Honorable George Miller
Ranking Member
Committee on Education and the Workforce
House of Representatives

The Honorable Lynn C. Woolsey
Ranking Member
Subcommittee on Workforce Protections
Committee on Education and the Workforce
House of Representatives

Appendix I: Objectives, Scope, and Methodology

To determine how long it takes the Occupational Safety and Health Administration (OSHA) to develop and issue safety and health standards, we reviewed occupational safety and health standards and substantive updates to those standards. We selected standards that met two criteria: (1) they were published as a final rule between calendar years 1981 and 2010 and (2) OSHA identified each standard as significant. To identify our universe of standards for this analysis, we first conducted an electronic legal database search for final rules published by OSHA in the *Federal Register* between 1981 and 2010. We chose this time frame because it spans multiple executive administrations and changes in congressional leadership. Also, several statutes, executive orders, and key court decisions affecting OSHA's standard-setting process became effective in or after 1980. We excluded from our review any rules that were not occupational safety or health standards, such as recordkeeping requirements or general administrative regulations,[1] and any rules that were minor or technical amendments to existing standards. For this list, we included only standards for which OSHA's semiannual regulatory agenda or other evidence indicated that OSHA considered the standard to be important or a priority, including but not limited to standards that met the definition of "significant" under Executive Order 12866. For each standard, we identified the dates of three regulatory benchmarks—initiation,[2] proposed rule, and final rule[3]—and calculated the time elapsed between each benchmark to analyze trends. We confirmed with OSHA staff the accuracy of our selected benchmark dates and that the list of standards met our criteria.

There are some limitations to this approach because the development of a standard may not have a clear beginning or end point. For example, OSHA may have begun work on a standard prior to its appearance on the regulatory agenda or the publication of a Request for Information or Advance Notice of Proposed Rulemaking in the *Federal Register*.

---

[1]In making this determination, we did not assess whether any particular rule met the definition of "occupational safety and health standard" under the OSH Act.

[2]For the purposes of this analysis, we considered a standard's initiation date to be the date OSHA publicly indicated starting work on the standard in the *Federal Register* by publishing a Request for Information or Advance Notice of Proposed Rulemaking. In cases where OSHA did not indicate in the final rule having published either type of notice, we used the date the standard first appeared on OSHA's semiannual regulatory agenda.

[3]For the purposes of this analysis, we considered a standard to be "finalized" on the date it was published in the *Federal Register* as a final rule.

Conversely, it is possible that although a standard appeared on the
regulatory agenda, work did not begin on the standard until sometime
later. According to OSHA officials, once development of a particular
standard has begun, work may stop and start again due to various factors
such as changing priorities. Furthermore, the date a final rule was
published does not necessarily coincide with the date the rule took effect,
which may be some time later. While our analysis will not reflect these
distinctions, we selected these benchmarks to ensure consistency and
maximize comparability across different standards.

To identify the key factors affecting OSHA's time frames for issuing
standards and ideas for improving OSHA's standard-setting process, we
conducted semistructured interviews with current and former Labor staff,
as well as occupational safety and health experts, and analyzed their
responses. We identified these experts, who represented both workers
and employers, through our own research and through recommendations
from other experts. The experts had direct experience with setting
standards at OSHA, testified at past congressional hearings on
occupational safety and health issues, or published written material on
federal rulemaking. Finally, we reviewed relevant federal laws,
regulations, executive orders, and other guidance and interviewed
officials from the Office of Management and Budget to determine the
required steps in the standard-setting process and how those
requirements affect the time it takes OSHA to develop and issue
standards.

To identify alternatives to the typical standard-setting process available
for OSHA to address urgent hazards, we reviewed relevant federal laws
and interviewed current OSHA staff and attorneys from the Department of
Labor's Office of the Solicitor. We also interviewed experts identified as
described above. We assessed the extent to which OSHA has used its
authority to issue emergency temporary standards by analyzing a history
of petitions for these standards provided to us by Labor staff.

To determine whether rulemaking at other regulatory agencies offers
insight into OSHA's challenges with setting standards, we explored the
regulatory process at three other federal regulatory agencies and offices.
For these comparisons, we selected agencies with authority to issue
regulations relating to public health or safety. We also included some
agencies whose statutory frameworks were similar to OSHA's and some
whose statutory frameworks were different than OSHA's. We based our
selection of comparison agencies and offices on our interviews with
experts, as well as a review of the literature, previous GAO work, and

relevant federal laws. Using these criteria, we initially selected Labor's
Mine Safety and Health Administration (MSHA) and two offices of the
Environmental Protection Agency (EPA): the Office of Pollution
Prevention and Toxics and the Office of Air and Radiation. For the EPA
offices, we specifically focused on their rulemaking experiences under
section 6 of the Toxic Substances Control Act and section 112 of the
Clean Air Act. However, after further review, we concluded that the Office
of Pollution Prevention and Toxics did not offer insights for OSHA
because of the office's limited recent standard-setting experience and, as
a result, we excluded the Toxic Substances Control Act from our review.
Through a review of relevant federal laws and semistructured interviews
with staff in EPA's Office of Air and Radiation and at MSHA, we learned
about challenges each agency faces when developing and issuing
regulations and the factors that affect their time frames. Although states
may also issue standards in the absence of an applicable federal
standard or under an OSHA-approved plan, we did not look to these
states to gain insight into OSHA's challenges with setting standards.
Based on our interviews with experts, and because rulemaking at the
state level is governed by state law and is not subject to federal
rulemaking procedural requirements, we determined that any
comparisons between OSHA and states with respect to time frames for
issuing standards would be inapt.

We compiled the ideas for improving OSHA's standard-setting process by
analyzing statements from interviews with current and former agency
officials and experts representing both workers and employers. The six
ideas discussed in the report represent those most frequently mentioned
that are not otherwise addressed by other parts of our report.

We conducted this performance audit from February 2011 to April 2012 in
accordance with generally accepted government auditing standards.
Those standards require that we plan and perform the audit to obtain
sufficient, appropriate evidence to provide a reasonable basis for our
findings and conclusions based on our audit objectives. We believe that
the evidence obtained provides a reasonable basis for our findings and
conclusion based on our audit objectives.

Table 2 presents a summary of federal rulemaking requirements that apply to OSHA standard setting. This table is not intended to be a complete list of all procedural requirements that govern rulemaking at OSHA or at other federal regulatory agencies. In addition, this table presents only a selected summary of the requirements; for the complete requirements contained in each source, refer directly to the cited source.

Table 2: Selected Procedural Requirements for Federal Rulemaking

Source of requirement	Year enacted or issued	Citation	Description of requirement
Paperwork Reduction Act of 1980	1980	Pub. L. No. 96-511, 94 Stat. 2812, codified as amended at 44 U.S.C. §§ 3501-20.	Agencies are required to publish for public comment any proposed collection of information associated with a proposed rule. Agencies must then submit the proposed information collection to the Office of Information and Regulatory Affairs, and certify that, among other things, the collection is necessary for the proper performance of agency functions, is not unnecessarily duplicative, and reduces burden on respondents to the extent practicable and appropriate. The information collection must inform respondents why the information is being collected, how the information will be used, and provide an estimate of the burden. The Office of Information and Regulatory Affairs must, after another public comment period, approve each information collection request and assign it a control number before it can be implemented.
Regulatory Flexibility Act	1980	Pub. L. No. 96-354, 94 Stat. 1164 (1980), codified as amended at 5 U.S.C. §§ 601-12.	Agencies are required to publish for public comment, along with the proposed rule, a regulatory flexibility analysis, or certify that the proposed rule would not have a "significant economic impact upon a substantial number of small entities." The regulatory flexibility analysis must contain, among other things, a description of the reasons for and objectives of the rule, a description and estimate of the impact of the proposed rule on small entities, and a description of potential alternatives that could minimize the impact on small entities. When publishing the final rule, the agency must also publish a final regulatory flexibility analysis, addressing the comments received and explaining why alternatives were rejected.
Executive Order 12866[a]	1993	58 Fed. Reg. 51,735 (Oct. 4, 1993).	Agencies are required to submit "significant" regulatory actions[b] to the Office of Information and Regulatory Affairs before publishing them in the Federal Register, including the text of the regulatory action, as well as the agency's assessment of its potential costs and benefits. For economically significant rules, the agency must also submit a cost-benefit analysis of the proposal and potential alternatives. Staff from this office generally must notify the agency of the results of its review within 90 calendar days of submission.
Small Business Regulatory Enforcement Fairness Act of 1996	1996	Pub. L. No. 104-121, tit. II, 110 Stat, 847, 857-74, codified in scattered sections of 5 U.S.C. and 15 U.S.C., and as a note to 5 U.S.C. § 601.	If a proposed rule is expected to have a significant impact on a substantial number of small entities, OSHA, EPA, and the Bureau of Consumer Financial Protection are required to work with the Small Business Administration to form panels with representatives of affected small businesses, prior to publishing the rule. Agency staff must publish the recommendations from panel members in the *Federal Register* along with the proposed rule.

Source of requirement	Year enacted or issued	Citation	Description of requirement
Congressional Review Act	1996	Pub. L. No. 104-121, § 251, 110 Stat. 847, 868-74 (1996), codified at 5 U.S.C. §§ 801-808.	Agencies are required to submit their rules to Congress and GAO before they can take effect. GAO must report to Congress on agencies' compliance with procedural requirements. Major rules[c] cannot be effective until 60 days after publication or submission to Congress, whichever is later. If Congress enacts a joint resolution of disapproval within a certain time period after a rule is submitted, the rule shall not take effect (or shall not continue in effect), and it may not be reissued in substantially the same form unless expressly authorized by subsequent law.
Information Quality Act	2000	Consolidated Appropriations Act, 2001, Pub. L. No. 106-554, § 515, 114 Stat. 2763A-153 to 2763A-154 (2000) (44 U.S.C. 3516 note).	The Office of Management and Budget and federal agencies are directed to issue guidelines for ensuring and maximizing "the quality, objectivity, utility, and integrity of information" agencies disseminate, including information that supports regulatory actions.[d]

Sources: GAO summary of selected federal laws and executive orders.

[a]Executive Order 13563, among other things, reaffirmed the principles, structures, and definitions established in Executive Order 12866. 76 Fed. Reg. 3821 (Jan. 21, 2011).

[b]A regulatory action is defined by Executive Order 12866 as "significant" if it will (1) have an annual effect on the economy of $100 million or more or adversely affect in a material way the economy, a sector of the economy, productivity, competition, jobs, the environment, public health or safety, or state, local, or tribal governments or communities (also called "economically significant"); (2) create a serious inconsistency or otherwise interfere with an action taken or planned by another agency; (3) materially alter the budgetary impact of entitlements, grants, user fees, or loan programs or the rights and obligations of the recipients; or (4) raise novel legal or policy issues arising out of legal mandates, the President's priorities, or the principles set forth in the executive order.

[c]A "major rule" is defined in the Congressional Review Act as a rule that the Office of Information and Regulatory Affairs finds has resulted in or is likely to result in (1) an annual effect on the economy of $100 million or more; (2) a major increase in costs or prices for consumers, individual industries, federal, state, or local government agencies, or geographic regions; or (3) significant adverse effects on competition, employment, investment, productivity, innovation, or on the ability of United States-based enterprises to compete with foreign-based enterprises in domestic and export markets.

[d]Office of Management and Budget guidelines issued pursuant to the Information Quality Act require agencies to conduct a peer review of certain scientific information. Information Quality Bulletin for Peer Review, 70 Fed. Reg. 2664 (Jan. 14, 2005).

Appendix III: Comments from the Department of Labor

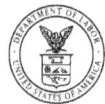

U.S. Department of Labor

Assistant Secretary for
Occupational Safety and Health
Washington, D.C. 20210

MAR 1 6 2012

Ms. Revae E. Moran, Director
Education, Workforce, and Income Security Issues
U.S. Government Accountability Office
441 G Street, N.W.
Washington, D.C. 20548

Dear Ms. Moran:

Thank you for the opportunity to comment on the Government Accountability Office's (GAO) proposed report entitled "Multiple Challenges Lengthen OSHA's Standard Setting." The Occupational Safety and Health Administration (OSHA) appreciates your detailed review of OSHA's rulemaking process and thorough analysis of the many hurdles faced by the agency when promulgating standards. Our response was prepared in collaboration with the Mine Safety and Health Administration (MSHA), who also reviewed the proposed report.

As the report states, Congress assigned to OSHA the authority and responsibility to issue occupational safety and health standards in order to protect the health and safety of 130 million workers, employed at more than 8 million U.S. worksites. The GAO's task in this report -- identifying and addressing the main causes for delay of OSHA standards – is an important and needed exercise. Preventable delays in issuing these important safeguards lead to the needless injury, illness and death of American workers. In its rule-making activities, OSHA is committed to issuing workplace safeguards that protect the health and safety of workers without imposing unnecessary burdens on employers. It is a challenging task to identify ways to speed the process of issuing these regulations, while continuing to provide abundant opportunities for stakeholder input.

OSHA agrees with GAO's recommendation to formalize the collaborative relationship between OSHA and NIOSH. In fact, NIOSH already routinely plays an integral part in the development of OSHA standards. For example, NIOSH performed technological feasibility assessments, risk assessments, and scientific investigations for several of the high-priority rulemakings including butadiene, methylene chloride, hexavalent chromium, silica, and diacetyl. We believe maintaining this relationship is critical for the viability of OSHA's regulatory program.

The GAO's recommendation represents one important step in the giant task of reforming the complex system that causes decades-long delays in issuing the standards on which workers' lives and health depend. GAO's report cites many other external factors that may also have a significant impact on the rulemaking process, including the effect that court decisions, executive orders, and legislative mandates have had on slowing the rulemaking process.

2

GAO has concluded the most time-consuming impediments to the promulgation of timely OSHA regulations are external to the agency and largely beyond the agency's control. The GAO consulted numerous experts who made several policy recommendations that, if implemented, would likely speed up the process of issuing worker protection standards without reducing the agency's responsibility to maintain the quality of standards, guarantee sufficient stakeholder input, and consider the potential regulatory burden on the economy. Such recommendations include expanding the use of voluntary consensus standards, statutory revisions establishing alternative feasibility assessment methods, and imposing statutory deadlines for standard setting through acts of Congress.

The GAO concluded that most of the suggestions recommended by experts for improving OSHA's standard setting process were largely outside of the agency's authority. Nevertheless, some of the ideas expressed by the experts as well as lessons learned from the diversity of laws that govern rulemaking at other agencies that issue quality regulations more rapidly than OSHA, should be strongly considered by those considering how the regulatory process can be made more responsive to the needs of worker safety and health.

Thank you for the opportunity to review and comment on the draft report.

Sincerely,

David Michaels, PhD, MPH

Appendix IV: Comments from the Department of Health and Human Services

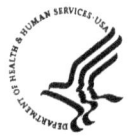

DEPARTMENT OF HEALTH & HUMAN SERVICES

OFFICE OF THE SECRETARY

Assistant Secretary for Legislation
Washington, DC 20201

MAR 0 9 2012

Revae Moran, Director
Education, Workforce, and Income Security Issues
U.S. Government Accountability Office
441 G Street NW
Washington, DC 20548

Dear Ms. Moran:

Attached are comments on the U.S. Government Accountability Office's (GAO) report entitled, "Workplace Safety and Health: OSHA Could Improve Standard Setting with Enhanced Coordination" (GAO-12-330).

The Department appreciates the opportunity to review this draft section of the report prior to publication.

Sincerely,

Jim R. Esquea
Assistant Secretary for Legislation

Attachment

**GENERAL COMMENTS OF THE DEPARTMENT OF HEALTH AND HUMAN
SERVICES (HHS) ON THE GOVERNMENT ACCOUNTABILITY OFFICE'S (GAO)
DRAFT REPORT ENTITLED, "WORKPLACE SAFETY AND HEALTH : OSHA
COULD IMPROVE STANDARD SETTING WITH ENHANCED COORDINATION
(GAO 12-330)**

NIOSH agrees with the GAO's recommendation of a more consistent collaboration between
NIOSH and OSHA on occupational hazard research so that OSHA can more effectively leverage
NIOSH expertise to determine the needs for new standards.

NIOSH has a memorandum of understanding (MOU) in place with OSHA that provides for data
sharing from OSHA's inspection database (IMIS) and NIOSH's blood lead database (ABLES).
NIOSH and OSHA also have a good working relationship that includes regular informal and
formal meetings between the NIOSH director and OSHA's assistant secretary, and a regular
conference call meeting of NIOSH-OSHA Liaison and Information Exchange (NOLIE) staff.
We agree with the GAO's recommendation that NIOSH and OSHA should establish a broad and
general MOU that provides for continued and regular interactions in the future

Appendix V: GAO Contact and Staff Acknowledgments

GAO Contact	Revae Moran, Director, (202) 512-7215 or moranr@gao.gov
Staff Acknowledgments	In addition to the individual named above, Gretta L. Goodwin, Assistant Director; Sara Pelton, Analyst-in-Charge; and Anna Bonelli, Analyst-in-Charge; managed all aspects of this assignment; Suzanne Rubins and Sarah Newman made significant contributions to all phases of the work; Sarah Cornetto made substantial contributions by providing legal advice and assistance; Jean McSween provided assistance in designing the study; Ashley McCall provided assistance with occupational safety and health literature; Kate van Gelder and Susan Aschoff assisted in message and report development; James Bennett created the report's graphics; and Ashanta Williams, Lise Levie, and Daniel S. Meyer reviewed the report to check the facts presented.